The Lesbian Love Companion

Also by Marny Hall, Ph.D.

THE LAVENDER COUCH:
*A Consumer's Guide to Psychotherapy
for Lesbians and Gay Men*

SEXUALITIES

The Lesbian Love Companion

How to Survive Everything from Heartthrob to Heartbreak

Marny Hall, Ph.D.

Illustrations by Jim Coughenour

HarperSanFrancisco
A Division of HarperCollinsPublishers

THE LESBIAN LOVE COMPANION: *How to Survive Everything from Heartthrob to Heartbreak.* Copyright © 1998 by Marny Hall, Ph.D. All rights reserved. Printed in the United States of America. No part of this book may be used or reproduced in any manner whatsoever without written permission except in the case of brief quotations embodied in critical articles and reviews. For information address HarperCollins Publishers, 10 East 53rd Street, New York, NY 10022.

HarperCollins Web Site: http://www.harpercollins.com

HarperCollins®, 📖®, and HarperSanFrancisco™ are trademarks of HarperCollins Publishers Inc.

FIRST EDITION

Library of Congress Cataloging-in-Publication Data

Hall, Marny.
   The lesbian love companion : how to survive everything from heartthrob to heartbreak / Marny Hall ; illustrated by Jim Coughenour.
      ISBN 0-06-251431-8 (pbk.)
      1. Lesbian couples.   2. Love.   3. Separation (Psychology).
   4. Interpersonal relations.   I. Title.
   HQ75.5.H35   1998
   305.48'9664—dc21   97-33290

98 99 00 01 02 RRD(H) 10 9 8 7 6 5 4 3 2 1

To
Scout, Scamp, Perky, Snipe,
Kamela, Leander, Mrs. Smiley,
and the Tasty Butterfish

Contents

Acknowledgments

First and foremost, my thanks go to the small army of dykes who shared their lives and loves with me. Their stories are the soul of this book. I want to thank Sarah Schulman, as well. I will always be indebted to her for providing the impetus for this book.

Heartfelt appreciation goes to the friends who supported and encouraged me and who lured me out for meals and hikes when I began to turn into a cyborg. For these much-needed infusions of human spirit, thanks to Jeanne Adleman, Jane Futcher, Nanette Gartrell, and Diana Russell.

Many thanks, as well, to my distant muse. Despite her demanding schedule, Liana Borghi found time to read earlier versions of my manuscript and fill in my theoretical lacunae.

Whenever I got stuck in a cyberwarp, Freda Ances came through with her special brand of mazeltech support.

Whether I needed to track down some obscure bit of dyke arcana or just have my spirits propped up for another day, I could always count on Karla Jay. She is a true-blue friend. Ditto for Karen Kerner. Her e-mails were just the right mix of juicy, cliterary dish, and "atta-girl" encouragement.

Esther Rothblum has been unstinting with advice, support, and resources. I am very grateful to her.

Thanks to Esther Landau, Joan Biren, and Terry Ryan for their title assistance and Judith Stelboum for numerous tips and Vickie Reed at the copy center for her great spirit.

Lauree Moss provided loving support and valuable information at critical junctures.

I am particularly indebted to Janja Lalich, talented editor and writer, for her valiant attempts to correct my excesses.

Special thanks to Charlotte Sheedy and Neeti Madan for their support in the early stages of the project, and to Caroline Pincus for later-stage hand-holding.

Bouquets to the members of my lesbigay support group—Arthur Atlas, JoAnn Loulan, Jack Morin, and Jan Zobel—for their rock solid support over the years.

Boundless gratitude to Susan Kennedy for her willingness to make our relationship the testing ground for many of the theories in the book. For this she deserves the highest award that Lesbian Nation can confer: the Lavender Heart. Parenthetically, she is also an editorial genius, a great lover, and an irresistible *bon vivante*.

Finally, I want to pay homage to a trio of ghosts. Thanks to M. Belish for teaching me everything I know, to Richard for hanging around and helping me through this project when he wanted to be in Deya with Dan, and to Jill, the first dyke (but certainly not the last) to break my heart, thereby setting me on a lifelong quest to solve the mysteries of lesbian love.

The Lesbian Love Companion

Introduction

Where did the passion go?
   Have I made a mistake?
Is it really over?

The questions sneak up in the dead of night or assault us in broad daylight—the questions we whisper to ourselves or hurl at the strangers who were once our lovers. And when silence is our only response, we seek out professionals who can solve our painful riddles. After all, therapists are *supposed* to have the answers.

A lesbian couples' counselor for years, I had learned my craft well. I knew when to console and when to confront, when to probe and when to shut up. I knew how to stop a fight, how to start a dialogue, and how to assign exercises that would be helpful even if partners didn't bother to do them. But when it came to the inevitable what-went-wrong questions . . . I hadn't a clue. After a painful breakup of my own, I decided it was time I found out.

In 1985 I began interviewing long-term couples about their recipes for longevity. And I kept interviewing them.

After ten years of tracking a handful of couples through good times and bad, breakups and new beginnings, the formula for permanent partnerships still remained elusive. But along the way, I found out something even more intriguing: lesbian couples are gifted storytellers. It was this storytelling ability, developed out of necessity in a straight and often hostile world, that strengthened these couples' partnerships.

It makes sense. If we don't tell our own thick-and-thin parables, no one else will. When times are hard, chances are no beloved aunt is going to take us aside and insist that if she and Uncle Jake could make it . . . well then, by damn, so could we! There are no legal documents in the desk to certify our unions, no romantic movies on TV that celebrate our love. There is no church, no community, no government, no timeless tradition to reinforce the story of our togetherness and continuity.

It's up to us to do it ourselves. And we do. We tell our stories with cards and flowers, with plans and promises, with private rituals and public ceremonies.

But, as every good storyteller knows, the course of true love never runs smoothly, and somewhere between once-upon-a-time and happily-ever-after something awful happens: perhaps a value clash congeals into a permanent power struggle; maybe a trusted friend turns into a new lover. In spite of best efforts, the struggle may prove too much for us. The relationship ends. But, oddly enough, the story goes on.

But now it takes another form. Happily-ever-after turns into she-done-me-wrong or, even more commonly, I-done-myself-wrong: I chose badly, moved in too quickly, was too much of a co. They are stories we know by heart. Why? Because we've all told them. Again and again.

What I came to realize during my ten-year quest was quite simple. The forever-after story is compelling, but we need more than one way to think about partnerships.

Most of us aren't going to stay with our first, second, or even third partners. And in the face of devastating change, storytellers don't suddenly stop telling stories. They come up with reasons—explanations for why things went wrong and ways to avoid future catastrophes. Unfortunately, our determination to do it better next time around may only set us up for a new round of rapture and rupture.

The ideal of the perfect (or perfectible) couple is great—if you happen to be a therapist or the author of a how-to book. For most of us, however, trying to become a lesbian poster couple is a disaster. It reduces our remarkable array of relationships to one pass/fail model and turns us into intimacy overachievers or abysmal failures.

But what if, in addition to forever-after (or failed-forever-after), we had plenty of alternative ways to view the inevitable ups and downs, the surprising twists and turns in our relationships? What if, for example, we could see the conflicts that ruffle our relationships as positive—evidence that the Dora Doormat in all of us has finally been able to stand up for herself? Or what if, instead of regarding a new attraction as the beginning of the end, we saw the arrival of *the other woman* as perfectly normal, an envoy from the outside world we may have been neglecting?

In this new way of viewing relationships, anything is possible. The old bugaboo "lack of commitment" can suddenly look like day-at-a-time wisdom, and even those heartbreak-ers—unwanted endings—can turn into new beginnings. And the best part is that such transformations are within reach. We don't even have to stretch our imaginations to make up such stories. The raw material is all around us.

Out of a history of invisibility and silence, lesbians have devised some of the most unique (and creative) ways of having relationships—ways that defy convention and some-times appear downright crazy. We are everywhere. And when it comes to loving, we are also everything: Sexual tourists and merger queens, bisexual dabblers and chat room Romeos, polymorphous perverts and permanently asexual partners. But whether we like our sex spicy or bland or not at all, whether we break up regularly or stay together for keeps, whether we are partnered or embedded in a sprawling network of friends and other lovers, one fact is clear: our love lives are just as diverse as we are. And try-ing to fit our unique rhythms into forever-after is rather like Cinderella's sisters trying to jam their toes into those dainty slippers. One-size-fits-all ends up fitting no one. Our rela-tionships need to be just as diverse as the other aspects of our lives.

This book won't tell you how to become a perfect couple. It won't tell you how to jump-start flagging passion or live happily ever after. Our attempts to achieve these goals have added to lesbians' already-ample supply of self-doubts.

But the chapters ahead *will* give you a detailed tour of relationship options. By providing concrete examples and simple, easy-to-follow steps, *The Lesbian Love Companion* will guide you out of the not-good-enough framework that, for far too long, has demonized our differences and created catastrophe out of change. The book does what marriage manuals and lesbian couples' guides have failed to do. It breaks the forever-after mold and helps lesbians—couples and singles, the eternally faithful and the easily sleazy—think about their lives and loves in novel and positive ways.

Marny Hall
San Francisco

Chapter 1

Solving the Partnership Puzzle

When a couple comes to therapy for the first time, I check for membership insignia: the leather or tweed, the tattoos or gold earrings, the buzz cut or blond bob that will tell me whether my new clients belong to the butch/femme club or the crone clan, the punk or professional tribe of Lesbian Nation. Yet, as revealing as these dyke markings may be, they fade into insignificance during breakups. At such times, there is only one detail that counts: one partner wants to stay in the relationship; the other wants to leave.

The new couple in my office is no exception. As soon as they sit down, one partner nods tersely at the other. At this signal, the second woman fidgets briefly and then, as though reading from an invisible cue card, tells me that they have decided to separate.

"*We* haven't decided anything," snorts her partner. "You've decided. Why don't you tell her the whole story?" Then she turns abruptly toward me. "She's leaving me for someone else."

The two had called earlier in the week for a mediation. There are photo albums, camping gear, mutual friends, a computer, a CD player, and an arthritic calico to somehow divide. But, I soon see, all these items are decoys. As long as the two women can't resolve any of their custody disputes, they can buy a little more time before the separation begins in earnest.

After an hour, our fruitless negotiations collapse into a portentous silence. Suddenly, the angry partner announces that there's one thing they won't have to divide. "It's all yours," she declares, as she retrieves an official-looking document from the recesses of her knapsack. Slowly and deliberately she tears up their domestic partnership certificate, hurling the shreds in her girlfriend's direction. Mesmerized, I watch as the sad confetti scatters above us and rains down. Having made her point, the aggrieved partner stands up and stalks out. Before following, her girlfriend gives me a despairing look.

I take a deep breath and look around. Scraps of paper are everywhere. The dismembered document has settled like snow over my rug, chair, and desk. I have to brush the remnants off my appointment book to read my notes for the rest of the afternoon:

one o'clock. Roxy and Max—Together six years; no sex after first; want to move to country and buy house but worried about sexless future together two o'clock. Jo Jo and Molly—No sex since Molly remembered stepfather molested her as child

three o'clock. Taylor and CJ—CJ hates vibrator, but Taylor needs it to come

four o'clock. Sue and Kesha—Kesha in love with her AA sponsor; wants to "open up" relationship

five o'clock. Casey and Terza—Breaking up; check on support networks

More fragments. Pieces that once upon a time fit snugly together.

And as of that morning, I could add my name to the grim roll call of sexual mismatches, ruptured commitments, and broken hearts. After months of mutual torture, otherwise known as "the growth process," my lover and I had finally called it quits. I could not tolerate her new lover; she could not give her up. During our final counseling session, my partner informed me she would move out by the end of the month.

Over the years I worked as a therapist, I had witnessed hundreds of lesbian couples at the same crossroads. Had watched helplessly as once-loving partners hurled recriminations, pulled off rings, canceled the future. And I had learned, through the uproar, to hear the rending sounds of hearts at the breaking point. It didn't matter who had initiated the leave-taking, who felt left behind. Neither partner escaped unscathed. Nor did it matter if their relationship had been serene or conflict riddled; didn't matter that the departing partner's new passion was probably doomed from the start. Once the breakup had gotten inscribed in the destiny column, there seemed to be no turning back.

Couple problems, like couples themselves, come in all shapes and sizes. But of all the woes plaguing lesbian partners, outside affairs seemed to generate the most rancor.

If one partner had fallen in love with someone new, my role was usually limited to damage control. If I could show that all those angry accusations were simply the public face of private grief, perhaps I could turn the tirades back into tears and, if I was lucky, salvage some goodwill. They would need it in the future. And if by some miracle the new affair lost steam, perhaps the original couple—shaken but still intact—could pick up the pieces and start over. Occasionally, such reconciliations occurred. But more often, partners ended up bitterly estranged for a time. If and when the exes finally made their peace with each other, usually neither wanted to "go backward." Perhaps they became distant acquaintances who exchanged perfunctory nods if they happened to bump into each other once a year in line at the local gay film festival, or perhaps they even became good friends and even occasional lovers. Rarely, however, did they become partners again.

Of course, this as-the-crow-flies account hardly does justice to the breakup variations: the crafty dodges and hairpin turns, the desperate plea bargaining and faux endings. By the time it happened to me personally, I had already witnessed every possible evasive maneuver in my office. Perhaps that was why—from the first moment my soon-to-be-ex and I sat down together on *our* therapist's couch—I had such a bad case of déjà vu. I felt like a coroner trying to grasp the finer points of respiration. I knew too well how futile such a lesson would prove in the end.

The night before our last couple's session, I dreamed that Erin and I were together again. Instead of my usual early morning misery, I woke up bathed in the glow of Camelot. As far as I and most of my couples clients were concerned, happy long-term partnerships were nothing more than that: vibrant dreams that dissolved in the morning light. But I also knew that, for a few couples, conjugal bliss was more than a mirage. A handful of partnerships *are* permanent. Some couples *do* stay together for decades. For a lifetime. Perhaps if I could figure out the secrets of those chosen few, I could make a *real* difference in the lives of my clients. And I could avoid the pain of another agonizing breakup.

The Camelot Couples

I first spotted Kirsten and Grace at a friend's graduation party. They caught my eye as they exchanged a meaningful look during a time-out from hors d'oeuvres duty. The mini-encounter had taken my breath away. Not because it was particularly erotic. It wasn't. But because in that magic moment, I glimpsed the intimacy usually reserved for dreams. When I asked the hostess about the pair, she laughed. "I know what you mean. They're always like that. And they've been together for more than a decade." My informant shrugged. "I don't know their secret, but they've obviously got one."

Later that week, I found them in the phone book, and, without giving myself a moment to reflect on my folly, I dialed their number. Kirsten's chirrupy hello was daunting. What now? Explain that I was a brokenhearted, burnt-out therapist in search of the elixir of happily forever-after? She would probably report me to the crank call division of the phone company. I managed to mumble that I had met her at my friend's party. She remembered me or at least pretended to. I was, I said, doing a research project on lesbian couples. I wondered whether she and Grace would be willing to meet with me for an hour or so. A long pause and then, "Well, what have we got to lose?" We made a date.

Kirsten and Grace knew of another couple I could interview. Through friends, I heard of several other marathon marriages. And so it went. Within a month, I had located four couples who had been together for at least a decade. And, along the way, each had faced plenty of challenges. All four had managed to weather outside affairs, homophobic families, job changes, sickness, and a variety of other tribulations guaranteed to shorten the longevity of all but the most committed partners. I couldn't yet quite make out the spires of Camelot rising above the San Francisco fog, but I was sure I was on the right path.

For the next ten years, I kept track of the four couples. Sometimes, when our paths crossed accidentally at a party or lesbian event, I would catch up informally. If too many months had elapsed since our last contact, I would phone and ask if we could get together. During these more formal meetings, I relied on my tape recorder to be my second set of ears.

Through it all, I believed I would find the secret of enduring lesbian relationships. I was sure some key, some code, some pattern would eventually emerge. Perhaps a theoretical hinge—some unique intersection of class and race and temperament that, by some miracle, added up to compatibility. Perhaps it would be a critical incident—infidelity or sickness, for example—that inoculated the partners against all future seismic shifts in their circumstances. Perhaps I would find that a series of turning points—the purchase of a house followed, for example, by a momentous birthday or the birth of a child—eventually culminated in a critical mass of stability.

But no pattern *did* emerge. These women's lives and loves simply refused to be shoehorned into any of my theoretical containers. To add to my frustration, the growing blizzard of transcribed pages began to overflow my file cabinet just as insistently as partnerships themselves were eluding all my theories. The whole project was about to turn into a monument to chaos theory, and then I got a call from Kirsten. Tearfully, she told me that she and Grace had broken up.

After Forever-After

For the first time since our initial contact a half dozen years before, I arranged to meet with Kirsten and Grace separately. And it was during the time I spent with each of them, sifting through the rubble of Camelot, that I found what I was looking for.

The first clue was a discrepancy: the ragged edges—the *before* and *after* versions of the relationship—simply didn't match. It was natural enough for two sparring partners to have different accounts of the ending. But the differences went beyond such face-saving attempts to seize the moral high ground. Each woman's postbreakup observations of the relationship diverged dramatically from ways she had described the relationship while it was in progress. In fact, the *before* and *after* versions bore so little resemblance to each other that it seemed as though two entirely different relationships were being described.

For starters, the *before* and *after* accounts of Kirsten and Grace's sex life didn't match. During our first meeting, they had described their X-rated honeymoon. Sounding a bit nostalgic, Kirsten explained, "I was really in lust." When I met with Kirsten after the breakup, she explained matter-of-factly, "I never felt passionate chemistry with Grace."

Kirsten and Grace's psychological bond, turned this way and that in the light of new understanding, also changed colors. Early on, they explained that Kirsten's tendency to think of Grace, who was eleven years older, as her mother had been troublesome in the beginning. But, both concurred, such leftover business had finally been resolved with the help of therapy. "Finally, I can see Grace clearly," Kirsten had assured me in our earlier meetings. Afterward, interviewed separately, both blamed the breakup on the unresolved mother-daughter dynamic. "Since she could never free herself from the idea that I was her mother, she had to free herself from me," Grace observed.

Even their cherished world of friends toppled off its axis after the breakup. *Before,* both had always described their community of intimates as indispensable, the epoxy that held them together during the times their relationship threatened to fray. *After,* Grace was blunt: "There was no

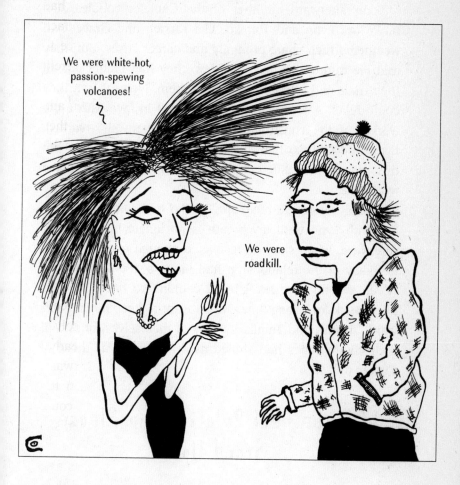

community. Not really." She claimed that it had all been a convincing mirage.

Soon afterward, another of the Camelot couples also broke up. Lynn and Tomiko, like Kirsten and Grace, had weathered their share of family and career crises. But, they told me during our first interview, they had finally put all their trials and tribulations behind them. Now, at last, they could relax. A few years later, Lynn fell in love with a co-worker at the construction company where she worked. Lynn and Tomiko had survived other outside affairs, but this time it was different. Lynn left. Tomiko thought she would die.

A year before the breakup, Tomiko had said, "I want to live with Lynn until my breath is no longer in my body." Afterward, when she had recovered enough to start dating, her view of the relationship had made a 180-degree turn: "Even if Lynn were available, I couldn't go back. We had been stuck for a long time. Now I want to keep moving forward." Lynn's and Tomiko's views of themselves, of sex, of their communities had shifted as dramatically as those of Kirsten and Grace.

Will the Real Relationship Please Stand Up?

The way in which these long-term couples rewrote their relationships after their breakups jogged my own memory. I remembered that I, too, had my *before* and *after* versions. During the time I had been with Erin, I had focused on the positives. Later, after any hope of reconciliation had passed, I put a different spin on the same events. Any friend I could buttonhole heard my postmortem: the relationship had always sucked. I was really lucky that Erin had found someone new. Otherwise, I might still be trying to turn myself into a pretzel to please her.

Of course, as a therapist, I had always counted on exactly such changing perspectives. Renouncing the past seemed to be part of clients' recovery. Hackneyed as it sounds, the best cure for broken hearts seemed to be the passage of time. But perhaps time does more than just heal old breakup wounds. Perhaps, I was beginning to see, even couples who stay together generate new versions of their relationships as they go. Suddenly the puzzle began to fit together.

I sifted through the transcripts of the two intact couples, looking for just such shifts in their accounts. And, sure enough, I found them.

Pat and Marie had been together longer than any of the other couples. And in more ways than one, they, too, had had their ups and downs. In fact, I first read about them in an article on lesbian rodeo champs.

When I first visited their horse ranch in southern California, I found them savoring some well-deserved rest and recreation. After vacillating for a year, Pat had finally ended an outside affair and decided, once and for all, to stay with Marie. She assured me that her wandering days were over. Permanently.

But when I visited them again a year later, Pat was embroiled in another liaison. And by then they had done some serious editing of their previous account. They "decided" that the apparent contentment they had been savoring when I first met them had been bogus. They both explained that underneath her deceptively calm exterior, Pat had been depressed and, consequently, vulnerable to the attentions of a bisexual co-worker.

I understood the need for such a revision. Without it, Pat would be branded as an incorrigible philanderer. But if Pat's behavior could be explained as somehow out of the ordinary—no matter how many times it happened—there was hope.

I found the same chameleon tendencies in the fourth relationship. Frieda and Salem were nonstop talkers, small business owners, and serious jocks who fell in love playing softball. And they, too, told me different truths at different times.

In the beginning of their relationship, they had carefully crafted a code of sexual conduct. Each was allowed to flirt with other women and even have extramarital flings. But serious involvement outside their relationship was taboo and honesty essential. When Frieda got emotionally entangled with another woman, she broke the couple's first rule. When she didn't admit it, she broke the second. Finally, she confessed. After a month of fireworks, both Frieda and Salem began to collaborate on a new version of events. They agreed that the new flame had simply satisfied Frieda's desire for a much-needed friendship, and they reclassified Frieda's "lie" about the new woman's significance. "Really," Salem told me earnestly, "it was just an omission on Frieda's part."

Lovers as Weavers

When the ground tilted under their feet, all four couples usually found ways to regain their equilibrium. Typically, the stabilizing force came in the form of a new revelation. Partners came to realize that domestic peace had really masked stagnation or vice versa, or that a sexual adventure really signaled a yearning for more commitment. Over the course of the decade I interviewed these couples, serious nesters turned into vamps and then back again into fierce guardians of the hearth. And for those who stayed together, painful ruptures metamorphosed into splendid new beginnings.

Finally I found the theoretical hinge I needed. And, as it turned out, it wasn't a hinge at all. Rather, it was a loom. Again and again, these couples managed to weave complex and confusing new circumstances into the ongoing stories of their durable partnerships. And during their years together, these women had become very adept at braiding seemingly incompatible threads into entirely new designs—designs that, depending on the circumstances, they might have to rip out and redo at any minute. On the other hand, I also sensed, underneath their capacity for rapid change, an old, unchanging pattern.

Part of the pattern of these women's lives had been firmly in place before they met—before, in fact, they were barely old enough to walk or talk. As little girls, each of these women had known she would grow up, find a mate, and live happily ever after. Though the gender of the prince had changed along the way, the story had remained the same.

But as far back as they could remember, each of these women had also prized solo adventures. These independent parts of their lives had nothing to do with finding a partner and settling down. Kirsten, for example, had always intended to undertake a solitary spiritual journey. Salem had always wanted to start her own business. Pat's lifelong goal had been to stay on a Brahma bull long enough to win the gold. However, not all of their adventures were so benign. Those that came unbidden—falling in love with someone new, for example—proved much harder to combine with their permanent partnerships.

When the new-passion strands of these women's lives clashed with the forever-after part of their designs, it took consummate skill on the part of both partners to harmonize all these disparate threads into a whole pattern. The durability of their relationships was a measure of their weaving skill. Take outside affairs, for example. If partners could somehow integrate "the other woman" into the ongoing couple's story, their relationship would continue. But if the affair could be perceived only as a betrayal, the partnership was doomed. But outside sex wasn't the only challenge for these weavers. Say two partners had an ongoing clash about whether or not to have children. If partners managed to make their continuing disagreement part of their ongoing couple's story, their relationship would continue. But if the conflict could be perceived only as an irreconcilable—and intolerable—difference, the relationship would probably end.

Once upon a Time

Storytelling helps couples at every stage. In the beginning, romantic stories about mysteriously crossed paths bonded and affirmed the new partners. For example, Frieda knew something special was going to happen at softball practice when Salem first threw her a ball: "When I caught it, it felt like it hit the most perfect place in the center of my being." The sparks started by the magical event have never stopped.

For Grace and Kirsten, the magic moment came when they were standing half naked on the edge of their campsite, brushing their teeth. "I knew right then and there," Grace reminisced, "that I wanted this woman more than anything."

Stationed in DaNang during the Vietnam War, Pat and Marie felt the earth move the first time they huddled together under the bed in Pat's hooch during an air raid.

Tomiko had fallen in love with Lynn at first sight. But it wasn't until they had slipped away from a church picnic, commandeered a rowboat, and spent the afternoon drifting, drifting over a sun-spangled lake that they knew they were meant to be together.

Besides framing their first encounters as special, the telling and retelling of stories about their relationships allowed the couples to weather crises. Faced with potentially hurtful or damaging revelations about themselves or their partnerships, all four couples uncovered previously hidden information—motives or memories—that, for a while at least, saved the day. In fact, it seemed that these relationships remained constant over long stretches simply *because* partners' accounts were constantly changing. Like shock absorbers, creative explanations cushioned and stabilized their relationships at those times when they threatened to unravel. And after the dissolution of two of the partnerships, new versions of "what really happened" helped the exes recover from broken hearts.

Much of what I did in therapy, I realized, was jump-starting couples' storytelling ability. Distressed partners came to counseling not because of any particular problems, but rather because their stories had been interrupted. If one partner had slept with someone else, for example, it was hard to keep believing—to convince each other—that theirs was a special relationship. But if I could pick up the threads of their ruptured story in a way that reconfirmed their lost specialness, I just might be able to restimulate their own storytelling. Instead of the standard interpretation of betrayal, for example, extramarital sex might simply mean something important about their own relationship. Unexpressed anger, perhaps, or the need for more freedom, which, censored or ignored, had appeared in the guise of an outside lover.

In short, it is not sex with a new partner, but the compromised storytelling ability of partners that ends relationships. When partners cannot tell their ongoing couples' stories in a way that can explain outside passions or boredom or conflict, they tend to go separate ways.

Of Queers and Quarks

Unfortunately, in our "just-the-facts, ma'am" world, storytelling has gotten a bad rap. Stories, we learn, are frivolous or just plain false, and the people who tell them are either con artists or grown-up children clinging to a make-believe world. And yet, as we all know, facts are never the pure data they pretend to be. A German scientist named Werner Heisenberg got a Nobel Prize for demonstrating the ways in which the observer always changes what is being observed. And though Heisenberg's Uncertainty Principle applied to subatomic particles, it is as true of queers as it is of quarks. In other words, there is no purely objective reality. In the process of perceiving the world, we always reinvent it; that is, we tell a story about it. Far from being a bad habit practiced by psychopaths and children, then, storytelling is our attempt to make sense of the disconnected fragments that come our way. One of Heisenberg's contemporaries, Norbert Wiener, summed up this all-too-human propensity nicely. The universe is nothing more, he wrote, than "a myriad of to-whom-it-may-concern messages."

New romantic partners excel at such storytelling. Straight or gay, new lovers seem to create private worlds out of details as trivial as the sound of a voice or the smell of a particular perfume. Unfortunately for lesbians, the celebrated troubadours of the twentieth century—from Puccini to Pope Paul, from Daryl Zanuck to Danielle Steel—amplify the stories of straight couples. Almost in self-defense, we must crank up the volume on our own epic tales of love and desire. We must be swept off our feet by tsunamis, melted into molten bliss by lightning bolts of lust. Our passions are so compelling, so our stories go, that we are willing to suffer oppression and ostracism in order to honor the truths of our bodies. But what happens if those truths change?

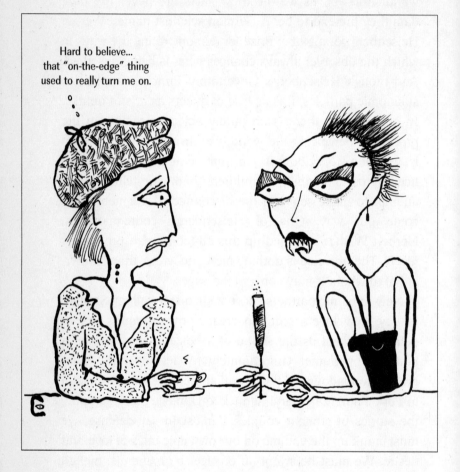

What if we no longer want sex with the partners to whom we have sworn lifelong devotion? Or worse, what if we fall passionately in love with someone new? What stories will we tell ourselves then?

At times, the four couples I interviewed, skewered on the horns of just such dilemmas, were forced to separate. Other times, though, by the brilliant twists and turns of their stories, they managed to escape into new realities that did not force a choice between cherished companions and new passions.

Lesbians and Bower Birds

The four couples I tracked for my research harvested the stories about their relationships from a wide range of sources. They had Hollywood to thank for their notions of true love and romance; Freud for the much-probed sunken continent of the subconscious; and fate for the cosmic encounters that studded their stories. They owed their butch/femme quotients to JoAnn Loulan; their quirks to astrology, and their "programming" to cybernetics. Their own checkered pasts, as well as their parents' relationships, had been rich in lessons in pitfalls to avoid. In fact, I found everything but the kitchen sink in these eight women's stories. And in one case, that was there, too—in the form of one couple's daily signature fight about whether it was clean or not.

There is a proverb in Tok Pisin, a New Guinean dialect, that is only half in jest: If you want to see what the world has to offer, just look at the bower bird's nest. Why? Well, the hodgepodge homes of these flying brigands are transistorized versions of everything around them. These birds heist whatever is not nailed down. Consequently, their chick nurseries are comprised of contraband as diverse as gum wrappers and fungi, plastic toothpicks and bits of cowrie shell polished by the ocean to a fine sheen. Like the bower bird, lesbian couples have a knack for "borrowing" an improbable array of nest-building materials. And like their avian doppelgänger, lesbian couples weave together all these bits and pieces, plus a zillion other improbable *objets trouvés*.

Yet, in spite of all their inventiveness, there was one bit of information missing from the four couples' stories. Since they hadn't occupied a fly-on-the-wall perch from which to observe themselves over the years, they didn't really know what superb Scheherazades they were. They were unaware of how convincingly they were able to reverse the direction of their tales, change their plots, introduce new character traits, or explain away new upheavals and dislocations.

But what if, just like the bits and pieces that lesbian partners have gathered from myriad other sources, the information about this storytelling talent was also added to our accounts of ourselves? Wouldn't we improvise with even more abandon? And wouldn't we trust ourselves to roam even farther and look in even more unlikely places for ways to embellish our narrative nests?

Discovered woven into one bower bird's nest was a fishing lure, an orchid (replaced by another as soon as it wilted), and a ruby missing from a distant temple Buddha. We, too, could use more exotic surprises, more curious twists and turns in our narrative nests, otherwise known as our love stories. For example, there may be new ways to tell the long-term-partner-versus-the-new-passion story that will bypass the usual either/or dilemma. Or perhaps in the process of telling old tales in fresh ways, we might be able to transform she-done-me-wrong dramas into heroic journeys that showcase our resilience and courage. If we understand the power of stories to change our lives, anything is possible.

This is a book about stories: about the forever-after fables that we know by heart and the never-before-told tales that spellbind us with their novel twists and turns. But most important, the book is about our own storytelling talent. The more we become conscious of our natural inclination to shape and reshape our lives with stories, the more we will be able to use our narrative gifts in purposeful and active ways.

Skillful storytelling is not always simple or easy. In fact, it takes nerve and courage to tell stories that differ radically from those being told all around us. Take loving women, for example. In order to become lesbians we had to love women. But we also had to tell stories about ourselves that contradicted all the previous myths that we had ever heard about who we were, about what was expected of us, about what was normal and right. And long after we declared ourselves dykes, we continue to tell against-the-grain stories.

For example, during a blustery night huddled around a campfire, we may swap coming-out stories with a group of backpacking buddies. Or maybe we reminisce with a lover about the bliss of that first cosmic kiss. Or perhaps we transform our private stories into public ceremonies that we perform in front of families and friends.

But even though we are constantly sharing the familiar classic, What It Means to Be a Dyke, with different audiences, telling such a puzzling and controversial story is not easy. It can be so challenging, in fact, that after a while we may feel as though we have done enough contrary storytelling to last a lifetime. We need a time-out. A recess. So we begin to coast. When it comes to other aspects of our lives and loves, we may simply chime in on the more conventional stories that we hear all around us every day. Yes, we are just like everybody else. Yes, we just want to find a mate, settle down, and start a family.

For many of us, echoing the conventional forever-after tale works well. Our partnerships do indeed last a lifetime. Others of us, however, might not fare so well. No matter how many times we tell the traditional one-and-only stories, they just don't seem to match our lives. But because we are master storytellers, we do what we do best: we start telling new tales about *why* the familiar formula isn't working. Unfortunately, these stories usually feature our own inadequacy: somehow we didn't do it right. We were too hasty; we moved in together too fast; we were too insecure. With a little bit of luck and a lot of therapy, we will do better the next time around.

But instead of dramas that feature our own failures, what if we told new stories—unconventional tales about novel relationships that go against the grain in the same way our lesbianism does? Wouldn't we be able to reshape the landscape of our lives and turn not-good-enough stories into rather remarkable accounts?

In order to tell such transformed and transformative tales, we need not trek to Borneo to retrieve rare orchids or hunt for rubies in the temples of Angkor Wat. We simply have to notice the treasures in our midst.

Adrienne Rich writes, "No one ever told us we had to study our lives, make of our lives a study." As soon as we do so, however, we notice something curious. All around us is the raw material for stories about love and life. We simply have to appreciate the dazzling array of intimacies already surrounding us. And before we can convert these relationships into valuable and triumphant tales, we have to believe that we are graceful and gifted storytellers who, no matter how hard it is, will continue to tell our strange and contrary stories.

Chapter 2

True-Life Love Stories: Creative Coupling Versus Forever-After

Let's start with the story we all know by heart. Forever-after is a tale that can wring a sigh or coax a tear out of the most hard-boiled dyke. The fable about lasting love has spellbinding power. And why shouldn't it? Commonplace as it is for many heterosexual couples, it is a tale of incredible privilege for lesbian couples. A dream come true after decades of deprivation—the interminable period when our only love stories had titles like *The Well of Loneliness* or *Women in the*

Shadows. Life was grim for pre-Stonewall dykes. Yet even in the days when our love was forbidden, we clung to tales of intrepid couples who survived—even thrived—in the wilderness: the hardscrabble adventures of Patience and Sarah, the madcap capers of Gertrude and Alice, the political passion of Del and Phyllis. Apparently with enough grit and wit, we could carve out our own secret oases. The story of love that is tough enough to survive in the middle of hostile territory has persisted even when our enemies have not.

Times have changed. The mainstream is no longer automatically off-limits to dykes. The old familiar taboos have changed shape or melted away. Come out of the closet, declare our true colors, and it's anybody guess what will happen next. Straight friends may rebuff us. Or, then again, they may confess their own secret same-sex fantasies. Our families may disown us. Or they may dance at our weddings. We can't be sure whether our adversaries will turn into allies or even if those old reliable allies, our lovers, will turn into strangers in front of our eyes.

In such a topsy-turvy world, the notion of till-death-do-us-part, dyke style, may have outlived its usefulness. In fact, tales of lesbian partners who overcome enormous odds to stay together are now more likely to prove harmful than helpful. Why is it that the love-triumphs-over-all stories that used to inspire us have turned into liabilities?

The Trouble with Forever-After

We know that lesbians come in more shapes and flavors than Ben and Jerry's ice cream. And most of the time, we don't lump ourselves together into a single race or class. Why, then, should one size fit all when it comes to romance?

It has always been difficult for the sluts and the curmudgeons, the solo travelers and the communally minded among us to live up to the gold standard of long-term couplehood. But today it's even more of a challenge. Now that the closet door has been ripped off its hinges and the light is flooding in, something no one had ever suspected is being exposed: women who love women have been hiding plenty of other secret selves. Suddenly single moms and cancer survivors, women of color and adult children of alcoholics, sadomasochists and bisexuals have made their debut. Even a few members of the Apple family have come tumbling out of the dark recesses. These parts of ourselves, and hundreds of others suppressed for the sake of peace in a confined area, have begun to demand their due: time, space, and respect. And these new demands haven't ended the moment we fall in love. Alliances with other members of our newfound clans frequently crisscross the once-sacred couple boundary, infringing on the intimacy previously reserved for our partnerships.

Even when they cause friction in our partnerships, these newly claimed identities are not about to be cowed into submission. There's no going back into the closet—any closet. And the more we or our partners try to deny or erase the freshly liberated aspects of our souls, the more our permanent partnerships are likely to turn into permanent power struggles.

The therapists who have stepped in to solve such problems haven't been much help. When the true-love story begins to show signs of wear and tear, they usually just modify the myth. Instead of the perfect couple, forever-after now features the perfectible couple. According to this updated version, when the going gets rough, partners should ferret out the personal insecurities that may be causing the problem. Or get some expert coaching on communication or sex.

When our efforts fail, we tend not to question the permanent partnership story. Instead, we conclude the failure of forever-after is our fault: we didn't work hard enough on the relationship. With only ourselves to blame, we do just that: ladle out the postbreakup guilt. We get a healthy portion. So do our ex-partners.

The only way we can redeem ourselves is to take the relationship test again. We vow to do better next time around. Be more cautious. Take things slower. In order to earn a passing score, we have to retrofit ourselves, find a new lover, and try again. Unfortunately, these resolutions to get it right don't improve the situation. In fact, they may even make it worse.

As a utopian fiction, the ideal of the perfect (or perfectible) couple is fine. But not in the real world. For the diverse dyke denizens of planet Earth, the old parables about pulling together may actually be pulling us apart—demonizing our differences and converting change into catastrophes. We need new stories—tales to instruct, to guide, to inspire us in changing times. And they are all around us. We just have to tune in and listen.

Lesbian Love Stories for the Changing Times

Lesbian relationships that last for decades probably fall into the same category as levitating or walking on water. After surviving troubles that would—and do—scuttle most relationships, such couples deserve all the recognition they can get. But, oddly enough, talking to women who have managed marathon relationships isn't necessarily the uplifting experience one might expect. Such accounts are brimming with love and companionship, but also they're often full of the same ennui, squabbles, disappointments, and sexual discord that scar heterosexual partnerships. After hearing about the conflicts that have simmered over the years, one can't help wonder if happily-ever-after might sometimes be a euphemism for unhappily-ever-after.

The Happily-Enough-for-a-Few-Years Love Story

What if we didn't view our lives through the rosy glasses of the ever-after-story-come-true? Might we notice that most of us have actually had a series of shorter relationships? And, furthermore, might we conclude that these two- or three- or four-year relationships have been very valuable to us?

LISSA AND BONNER

When Lissa and Bonner called it quits the day before their fourth anniversary, none of their friends could believe it.

Lis and Bon could hardly believe it themselves. To be sure,
they had their share of bad times—short-fused stretches
that they usually attributed to PMS. *But after a few*
slammed doors, the fights ended as abruptly as they had
begun. And the good times had far outweighed the bad.
An extralong honeymoon that had faded imperceptibly
into a more subdued pattern of maintenance sex. There
had been long bike trips every summer and, in the winter,
ski weekends with a gaggle of nieces and nephews. It was,
they both agreed, a good match. Too good to give up
easily. After Bonner fell in love with a co-worker, they tried
hard to make it work. But they couldn't. Now, a year after
a difficult breakup, both are relieved. They had settled
into a routine that had been comfortable enough, but as
they think back, the relationship lacked a certain spark.
Both agree that after the two-year mark, they probably
made better friends than lovers. Now, both embarking on
new relationships, each feels more alive than she has in
years. And the surprise happy ending: they are still in
each other's lives.

Lesbians have been members of a card-carrying subcul-
ture for half a century or so—long enough to be poked,
probed, and dissected by curious researchers. And, in fact,
in the past twenty years dozens of sociologists, anthropologists, and psychologists—often lesbians themselves—have
tracked our mating habits. Survey after survey produces the
same results: the average lesbian relationship lasts between
two and four years. Most lesbians do not stay with their
first, second, or even third lover.

In retrospect, breakups are not the tragedies they first seem to be. Inconsolable and brokenhearted partners seem to recover. As more time passes, most begin to feel lucky to be out of the very relationships that they once prized more than life itself.

Skeptical that ex-lover relief could be as heartfelt and widespread as it seemed, I decided to conduct some informal polls. From time to time, when I am giving a talk to a group of lesbians, I ask members of the audience to raise a hand if they can remember at least one unwanted breakup—some long-past parting in which they were an unwilling participant. Almost everybody's arm shoots up. Next, I ask, "How many of you would go back to that relationship if you could?" There might be one or two lone rangers who respond in the affirmative, but typically the only response is laughter at such a ludicrous proposition.

When we look back, most of us are terribly grateful that, despite the initial pain of separation, we are no longer with girlfriend #1, 2, or 3. Breakups may be tragic endings. But they are also valuable new beginnings—a necessary way to puncture some of love's illusions.

Scratch the surface of a grand passion, and oddly enough, we may even find its opposite: dispassionate, even disparaging feelings we harbor about ourselves. If a lover who is so ideal, so much wittier or prettier, returns our interest, we tell ourselves we can't be all that bad. Our self-doubts papered over, we coast until breakup time. Then a partner's departure only confirms what we suspected all along: unattractive and unlovable, we were only temporarily on sabbatical from dweebhood.

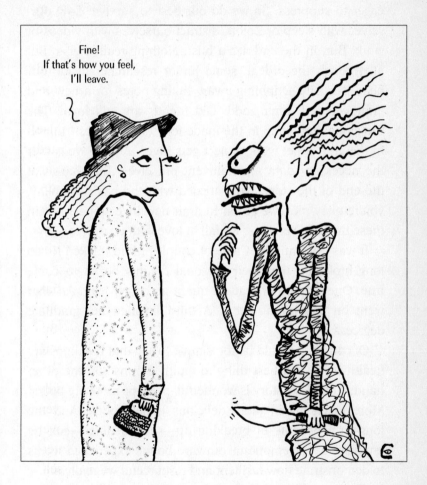

It's a devastating one-two punch: just as we're losing our lover, we are reuniting with the self-doubts we had been so eager to suppress. So we do our best to survive: drug ourselves with sleep or Zoloft, distract ourselves with videos or work. But, in the end, it's a bust. Nothing really helps. But all through the ordeal, some junior researcher inside our head is busily scribbling away. Taking notes for a new and improved self: hmm, odd. Old friends are still loyal. The brokenhearted klutz in the made-for-TV movie *does* triumph in the end. A pet work project gets raves. And so we gather the necessary data and reinvent ourselves. But that's not the end of the story. Not satisfied with the basic I'm-okay, you're-okay plot, we go on to draft new love stories. But in these updated versions, we fall in love with ourselves.

It was not until the Camelot couples I had tracked for so long broke up that their personal dreams began to come true. One ex-partner made a quantum career leap. Another went on a spiritual quest. A third finished her graduate degree.

Of course, it would be too simple to say that breakups are healthy, the next best thing to multivitamins. On the other hand, if one love story is wonderful, perhaps more are better. More lovers mean more delicious honeymoons. And the long-term benefits of breaking up—several times—can be impressive. The emotional outward-bound experience seems to demonstrate how resilient and resourceful we really are.

The Happily-Enough-for-a-Few-Years Love Story can be a useful addition to our romantic repertoires. If we have it on hand when we need it, it can give us a breather from the self-blame that so often accompanies breakups. It also helps us cherish the unique and shape-shifting intimacies we *do* have.

And, a surprising postscript: breakups create community. Think about it: the more times we break up, the more ex-lovers we create. The more ex-lovers, the more our chances that some of them eventually turn into "family"—beyond-friend, beyond-lover relationships that, having endured bitter breakups, will survive anything. Some ex-lovers become the long-term partners you can't leave even if you wanted to.

The Niche Love Story

Yet another new love story concerns time-managed romance. You might call it the story of niche love.

The first clue that a fast-track style of love has evolved to fit the new world of shrinking time and multiplying commitments is that our love, once etched in a locket or a valentine, is more likely to appear in an appointment book or electronic calendar. Squeezed in between work and play, between the friends and family sections in our pie-chart lives, is that old familiar heart. Condensed—perhaps even computerized—it is still visible.

KELLOGG AND SHANNON

It looks like a match made in hell. Kellogg is almost twice as old as Shannon and, as a business owner, earns ten times as much as Shannon ekes out as a vet assistant. But that's only the beginning of the incompatibilities that would jinx any other relationship. Kellogg is allergic

*to animal hair. Shannon always has a houseful of stray
cats she has rescued. Kellogg, a semicloseted Republican,
describes herself as being only slightly left of Attila the
Hun. Shannon, who identifies herself as a "vulgar
Marxist," is busily organizing a local cell of the Lesbian
Avengers. Even though the two women's schedules overlap even less than their interests, the two have managed
to carve out interludes: occasional overnights out of
town, or sushi and hot sex at midnight. After four years
of stolen moments, they're still in love. And their unconventional love affair has outlasted the partnerships of
friends who were full of dire predictions when Kellogg
and Shannon first got together.*

In the old love story, lovers met, dated, had sex, moved
in, and settled down. (The rumor about the U-Haul on the
second date is unfounded. According to a recent study, lesbians don't get serious about moving in until the fifth date.)
Niche Love scrambles the old sequence. Instead of the as-
the-crow-flies progression from meeting to marriage, the
new story moves backward. After the U-Haul urge has
peaked and subsided, the real dating begins. Weekend rendezvous. E-mail intimacy. Forget forever-after. Lovers will be
lucky if they can plan a getaway weekend.

The enemies of the new love story are also different.
Instead of the homophobic hordes of yesteryear, or even the
conniving Other Woman, the new villains 'r' us—our own
rapidly multiplying options and wildly proliferating obliga-
tions. Overbooked schedules require a new set of defensive
strategies. Instead of the courage necessary to keep a hos-

tile world at bay, our new circumstances demand nothing less than a black belt in social aikido. And these new equilibrium maintenance skills must be combined with the stealth of thieves. Lovers must become coconspirators, highwaywomen who steal interludes from an ever-intrusive, overly friendly world.

We've always lived and loved on the edges. But before, such uncharted borderlands were social margins, the places beyond the reach of convention. Now we have to contend with a new brand of marginality. We must find a way to tell our stories on the very edge of time itself.

The Sperm and Egg Mixer

Still another new story concerns a different kind of on-the-edge love. In this particular tale, the margin is disguised as the mainstream.

SHEILA AND DAVID

Sheila had met David at an introductory mixer for lesbians who wanted kids and gay men who were interested in being potential sperm donors. Within ten minutes after they met, the two of them decided they were identical twins who had somehow been separated at birth. There was no other way to account for the uncanny parallels in their lives.

David had grown up in Brooklyn, Sheila in Queens. Both had been red diaper babies, who, like their parents, had intended to make the world a better place to live.

Instead, each had ended up slogging through medical school. As soon as they had graduated, they felt free to come out. A decade later, in established practices, they both wanted kids.

It was a match so perfect it was almost too good to be true. And the more time they spent together, the more they liked each other. Really liked each other. So much so that when Sheila failed to get pregnant with the turkey baster approach, they decided to try the more traditional method. Sheila still didn't get pregnant. But something far more improbable happened. She enjoyed herself.

Checked the "normal" side of the moral boundary lately? Straights, of course, and now even lesbians—with their Hondas and their houses in the burbs—qualify as stable couples. It's much harder to see through the murk on the other side of the moral Maginot. So mysterious, in fact, are the inhabitants of the new abnormal turf that most of the time the language to describe them doesn't even exist. (What do you call a lesbian who has slept with a man? A byke?) Or when these boundary crossings *are* discussed, it is in codes barely intelligible even to the initiated.

The fresh crop of deviants and the new "mainstream" have it out every week in the personal columns of urban gay and lesbian newspapers. Ads proclaiming "nice normal girl" and "financially stable" spar for space with "Tranny seeking same" and "Boy dyke looking for daddy."

Most of us shake our heads, trying to puzzle out what radical sex practices the latest set of initials could possibly signify—what secret loves dare not speak their names to

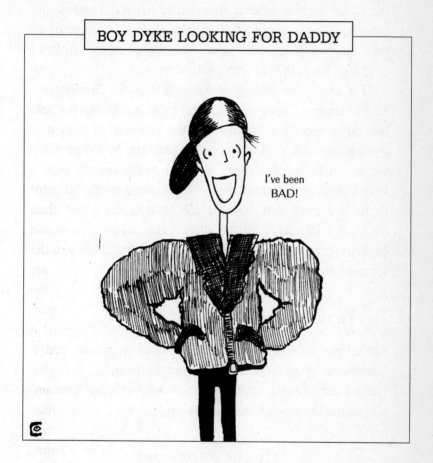

"normal" dykes, let alone straights. Our new love stories feature unlikely, and forbidden, attractions: not just the tattooed perv bowled over by the bi with the pierced clit, but the fierce feminist who is attracted to her p.i. nemesis, the s/m top. Or the two M-to-F transsexuals who, meeting in their support group for "newly straight women," fall head over high heels in love with each other.

This crossover gallery of Montagues and Capulets (or Montulets and Capagues) may not be to our liking; yet, just like our foremothers' forays into the verboten of their day, these stories are vital as boundary markers. In a time when we are in as much danger of being swallowed up by the mainstream as we are of being disappeared by the militant Right, we need our transgressive storytellers more than ever—as reminders that the silence exacted as a condition of belonging can be just as lethal as the deathly quiet imposed by the most virulent homophobe.

The Virtual Love Story

Sometimes we tell our subversive stories in private codes, sometimes by untoward deeds. And sometimes the underground conduits we seek out to tell our forbidden love stories shape the very tales we are telling.

TINA AND LORRAINE

They met on Sistanet@family.com. Both queer studies students, they felt adrift and isolated in a pale sea of classmates and teachers. Even their respective girl-

friends, though well meaning, were white. Whiter than white. "Women of pallor," Tina called them.

They began by flirting. Nothing serious. Light banter. Showing off. Name-dropping obscure authors and quoting memorable passages. Then they really started talking. About the state of their souls. They never declared their passion for each other. There was no point in stating the obvious, and anyway, what would they have said? 'Til death do us sign off?

Instead, they wrote each other an exotic love story in relays. Tina had them canoeing up the Amazon. Lorraine retorted with a stroll through Montparnasse. They camped out in Senegal, swam in the Aegean, and scaled Fujiyama. And the episodes always ended the same way. Lost in some world of their own making, they would begin to make love—to use each other's hands, lips, tongues as the guidebooks for the next, most intimate leg of their collaborative journey.

Long before the advent of cyberspace, lesbian love found a way to circumvent the roadblocks thrown up by the hard world. Respectable married ladies of the eighteenth and nineteenth centuries had a habit of writing impassioned, if sexually ambiguous, letters to each other. Though less flowery, and more to the point, the correspondence of their twentieth-century counterparts is equally passionate. One long-term partner interviewed in a survey of lesbian couples remembers, "We first said we loved each other after we had been writing. I asked her, 'Is it possible to fall in love with someone through the mail?'"

Sometimes, even partners who have no obvious reason to limit their passions to the page or the screen also practice the art of erotic extrasensory perception. In her autobiography *Lily Briscoe: A Self-Portrait,* lesbian author and artist Mary Meigs describes a similar nongenital form of ecstasy: "While my soul fainted with joy and my body quivered . . . [we] would build an airy pleasure dome for weeks and months, without the intensity and obligation of sex; there were no letdowns, only a sustained state of bliss."

Sometime or other, the necessity for secrecy has probably forced us to confine our passions to rapturous gazes and ardent whispers or flowery phases on perfumed stationery. All of our time and practice with disembodied love has served us well. We now possess a skill honed by necessity, and the new world—or at least the parallel universe offered by cyberspace—is ours.

In a piece called "Cyberdykes," Lisa Haskel writes, "In my new citizenship, I have no body, no voice, no location. . . . I'm light and magic." The Net is the perfect medium for the no-hands talent developed during years of repression. Also the perfect setting for dalliances. Flirtations, extramarital intimacy, and erotically charged musings with sudden soul mates a hemisphere away—off-limits if they occurred offline—are at our fingertips. And these affairs can be as compelling as any we might experience in the "real" world. We have gotten so good at touching without touching that we have turned absence itself into an exquisite pleasure. In the process, we have transformed online intimacy into a new love story.

The Companionable Love Story

Online or off, sex seems to be an indispensable part of our permanent partnership stories. But what if we add yet another tale to our growing repertoire? What if, right along with all the stories about off-the-beaten-path passions, we start telling the saga of long-term lesbian couples who are happy together *sans* sex? How might such a story go?

WIN AND NINA

Five years after they stopped having sex, Win and Nina still consider themselves a couple. And they act like one. They live and sleep together, and three years ago when Nina got the urge to leave Chicago and move to Seattle, they both took it for granted that Win would come along. Since then, they've spent a summer backpacking around the Northwest, started a kayaking business, and adopted two mutts.

There have been some dicey moments. The first time Win got a crush on a friend, they almost broke up. But after plenty of soul searching and a couples therapy session, they opted to stay put. "Now," Nina announces, "just to be safe, we have sex once a year."

"Yeah," Win adds, grinning, "on our anniversary. Whether we want to or not."

They don't regret their decision to stay together. Both claim they have what they want: a secure home life with a companionable mate. What they are missing, happily, is the old rapture/rupture two-step, the serial monogamy shuffle they did for so many years before they got together.

In 1983 *American Couples*, the largest survey of couples ever conducted, was published. The finding: after two years together, lesbians have significantly less sex than their gay male or heterosexual couple counterparts. Psychologists claimed women's socialization was to blame for the posthoneymoon plunge. Trained from birth to focus on the needs of others, a female partner could easily lose herself in close relationships. When two women get together, they doubled the possibility of such fusion. According to the sexperts of the day, too much closeness created a greenhouse effect that stifled passion.

Determined to remedy the mergers that rendered sex redundant, couples therapists assigned a variety of boundary-bolstering exercises. But try as they might to establish more separateness, plenty of their lesbian clients continued to prefer intimate tête-à-têtes and cuddling to sex.

Judging by the findings of successive surveys, the collective efforts of the therapists to stamp out lesbian bed death have failed. Lesbians in long-term relationships are still having less sex than women with men, or men with men. Much less. And though it hasn't been measured, lesbian couples are probably doing a lot more other things. Talking, for example, or touching in nongenital ways. But so long as genital touching continues to be considered an essential ingredient in long-term relationships, lesbians will be spending a lot of their intimate time worrying about the absence of sex or fighting about whether or not to do "it."

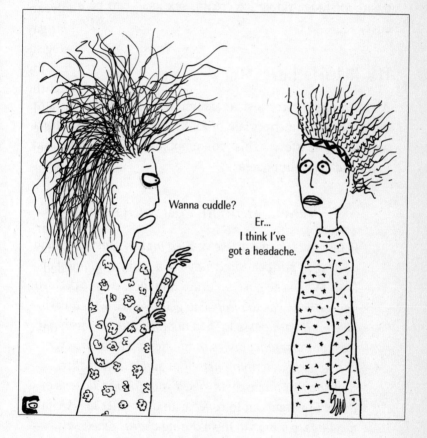

Sex *is not* the sine qua non of close relationships. Some of us may want sex in our lives. For others, it has always been a bothersome business at best. In our new love story, sex can take its rightful place: like a yen to try s/m or a desire for fudge ripple ice cream, sex itself can be a preference.

The Multiple Love Story

Another preference, just as common among lesbians as a desire for double chocolate *or* kinky sex, is the basis for yet another love story. This contemporary tale features an entire gallery of intimates.

TRAVIS AND THE COMMUNITY

Before she became a Twelve-Step junkie, Travis had had a string of partners stretching back to the beginning of time. When she gave up drugs and alcohol, she decided her sobriety was too fragile to get involved with a new lover. A month passed. Then another. Still no lovers. At least not permanent ones. And after a partner-free year she stopped describing herself as single. She realized that she was intensely involved with friends, dozens of them. She went out to coffee with them after her AA meetings, sat next to them during chorus rehearsals, and worked with them on fund-raisers. Once, when someone asked her if she was lonely, she burst out laughing. Never before had she been so close to so many women.

Lesbian theorist Teresa de Lauretis puts her finger on the problem of the invisibility of unpartnered lesbians when she writes, "It takes two women to make one lesbian." Minus a partner, we are also minus an identity. The moment we couple, however, we come alive. Our DNA unfurls, our lungs pump, and our hearts beat (in unison).

As a result of the two-equals-one bias (called the "cult of two" by one determinedly single friend), our love stories rarely feature unpartnered women. If they appear at all, it is only as phantoms: brokenhearted leftovers from past partnerships or the embryonic halves of future couples. Yet, in spite of the fact that so-called single women are invisible, they are often engaged in significant intimacies.

In these worldly romances, the standard ending never materializes. Instead of running off into the sunset with a lover, these women start businesses together or organize picket lines. They co-chair meetings and sit on the boards of nonprofit agencies. And along the way, these like-minded accomplices build bonds that rival more conventional passions.

In the process of pursuing our dreams, many of us form tight relationships. Such collaborative intimacies differ from erotic passions or even supportive friendships, though often they can and do have elements of both.

The two lesbian cofounders of a software company recall that when they first met, there was a certain frisson between them that could have developed erotically. But if they got involved sexually, they were afraid they would jeopardize what they *did* have. One of the partners searches for the words to pinpoint their brand of magic: "It's like finding a playmate who plays the same way you do and knows the same things you know." Her partner echoes her sentiments: "It is wonderful to be able to relate to each other in a way that we cannot relate to anyone else. We know what we're going to say without finishing sentences. We make leaps that border on the telepathic."

Besides being satisfying and supportive, these linkups are valuable for another reason: such associations defy easy classification. What exactly are these collaborators to each other? Sisters? Soul mates? Co-adventurers? Nothing quite fits. All we know for sure is that they have managed to bypass the traditional forms of togetherness and set out with improbable companions for we know not where.

Such shape-shifting intimacies compete with traditional love stories. And yet, in certain instances they may also help preserve them. How? At one time or another many of us are faced with an excruciating dilemma: a choice between a new passion and a cherished, permanent partner. The more we can generate alternative stories about in-between intimacies that cannot be pigeonholed, the less likely we are to retell the tired old either/or story about a forced choice between bitter rivals.

Each of our passions is different. Each deserves its own niche and its own story. Boldly, without apology, we need to begin to sketch our diverse intimacies—to tell our love stories to ourselves, to our partners, and to the world at large.

Couples may or may not break up. But the old love story has fractured into a profusion of new stories ready to be told: tales of brief encounters and serial monogamy; of uncoupled couples and part-time lovers; sagas of Boston marriages and merger queens, of open relationships and secret affairs; stories about passionate collaborations and marriages of convenience. About lovers separated by continents and close as a keyboard.

Using our own private languages and signal events, we are going to have to tell our real love stories. Not picture-perfect partnerships, but what *is:* everyday intimacies that are ordinary and messy, verboten and improbable. And after we have crafted our stories from our separations and reunions, our wartimes and peacetimes, our sacred moments and special observances, we need to broadcast them loud enough so they can be heard above the insistent claims of the forever-after story. We have to learn to listen to and speak our own poetry, no matter how contrary it may sound.

Chapter 3

Recovering from the Bruiser Breakup: A Revolutionary Remedy

Happily ever after is . . . well . . . a *happy* tale. But it is also a bit of a bully. Its refrain, crooned or strummed relentlessly on every pop station and performed in every cinema, effectively silences more subtle or contrary chronicles. Yet there is one story that the blissful fairy tale doesn't drown out. In fact, this story, entitled the Bruiser Breakup, seems to go hand in hand with true romance.

I'm sure there is such a thing as an easy breakup: a situation where one day, during a pleasant stroll on the beach, both partners agree in a relaxed, rancor-free way to go their separate ways. But as plausible, as desirable, as such a scenario might seem, our breakups are rarely straightforward or easy. Unfortunately, for the believers in forever-after, there are no sensible decisions to separate, no amicable partings. Only one finale is possible: if and only if one partner's betrayal is too monstrous to forgive can the other leave. But usually not peaceably and not right away. In other words, the only choice facing disillusioned partners is not whether to stay or leave, but whether their breakup will consist of a epithet-hurling jihad or a long journey through gulag iciness.

The evil twin of the romantic fairy tale is a she-done-me-wrong drama, an emotional *grand guignol* that features grisly discoveries and epic betrayals, tattered promises and shattered hearts. Eventually, ex-lovers recover. But not for a long time and not entirely. Years after the breakup, the survivors of such ordeals still show signs of trauma.

The evidence of breakup trauma is apparent even when couples come to therapy for minor problems: Say, for example, one partner complains that her lover goes ballistic whenever she is a minute late. When I poke around a little in the history of the short-fused member of the couple, I find that one day, without any forewarning, her previous partner didn't come home at all. Instead, she called to announce she had met someone new and that she would be coming by to pick up her things that weekend.

Or say anxiety about lesbian bed death has brought the couple in. One partner begins to hound the other if she feels that too many days have elapsed since the last time they made love. When I ask the worried partner about her experience with past lovers, she informs me the drop in sex "was always the beginning of the end" in her past relationships.

It doesn't matter what the partner friction is about. All too frequently a momentous breakup (or two or three) seems to be at the bottom of it. Although long past, a painful separation is nevertheless the real culprit behind the present-day problems the couple are so concerned about.

The Microbreakup Remedy

Most of us are terrified of the prospect of suffering through another Big One. So, in an effort to make partnerships permanent, we pile on the dos and don'ts. But such rupture-proofing strategies may backfire. More rules and regs may only mean more rugs to pull out from underneath the relationship at some point down the road.

There is another, much simpler remedy for postbreakup trauma: if we start to pay attention to nontraumatic breakups—the little separations and ruptures that are normal parts of our everyday lives—we will notice that all partings don't signal the End. In fact, the very opposite is true: most separations lead to reunions. And comings and goings are the very heartbeat of our partnerships.

Just like love stories, breakups come in all shapes and sizes. From large to little, total to partial: everything from daily interruptions to permanent separations. Obviously the big ones, like death and divorce, become permanent memories. They also become epic tales: My First Broken Heart sits on the shelf right next to such classics as My Coming-Out Story or Lesbo Lust Part 1.

Chances are other breakups—unnamed and therefore unnoticed—never make it into our personal registers of important events. Yet if we've been with a lover beyond the honeymoon stage, ruptures have probably become as commonplace as raptures. And whether such interruptions are accidental or intentional, secret or loudly proclaimed, they aren't fatal to us or the relationship. In fact, far from signaling the end, small breakups even strengthen our intimacies.

In a paradoxical way, the breakups that punctuate our daily lives bond partners. When we perceive a threat to our intimacy, most of us respond in a predictable way: we produce a sudden flurry of pet names or special acknowledgments or resolutions to be more considerate next time. In our own private language, we tell a story that goes something like this: we have problems for sure. Who doesn't? But we're committed enough to hang in there when times get tough. We've proven, over and over, that we are still very special to each other.

Breaking Up the Breakup Story

Unfortunately, because of fear of breakups, we automatically try to avoid or deny such small breakups, those very interruptions, disappointments, losses, and separations that toughen our intimacies. If we start to name and notice these small breakups, we can add a new story to our repertoire: the No Biggie Breakup. The more NBBS we can tell, the more we will be able to reduce the anxiety about the going-away part of the coming and going that comprises intimacy.

The following examples of NBBS break up the breakup story into a profusion of smaller tales: stories of accidental time-outs and psychological ruptures, chance interruptions and intentional sabbaticals.

The Accidental Breakup

KATE AND STEPH

Occasionally Kate would snore. Zzzz's loud enough to wake up Steph, who would, in turn, toss and harrumph until Kate woke up. And there they would be, both wide awake, listening to their upstairs neighbor practice her salsa steps or worrying about how little sleep they were getting. On the mornings after these episodes, both felt as though they had just camped out at a wild animal park. Still, the prospect of getting out of bed at 3:00 A.M. and unfurling a chilly sleeping bag in another room seemed infinitely worse. So they endured the occasional bout of interrupted sleep. Then, one night during a marathon video session, they both fell asleep on the living room couch. When Kate started snoring, Steph woke up, covered Kate with a blanket, and crawled back into their bed. Except for an occasional weekend spent with family, it was the first time they had slept apart since they had been together.

When we take a closer look at the presumed opposite of breakups and magnify to the tenth or hundredth power the daily events in the lives of stable committed couples, we find something surprising. Instead of long unruffled stretches of togetherness, our partnerships turn into a web of hairline fractures. Our closeness is interrupted when we go to work in the morning or fall asleep at night, when we opt to spend the evening out with a friend or withdraw to our room in a private funk. Even events that celebrate togetherness can suggest separation. An anniversary party that quantifies our shared time also intimates that the accumulation of years cannot continue indefinitely.

Intimacy requires just such daily punctuation. In the same way that our immune systems produce particular anti-bodies at the first sign of alien microorganisms, the small fissures that appear in our bonds cause us to reaffirm our partnerships. We will tell little tales of our togetherness with extra hugs or promises, phone calls or cards.

The Virtual Breakup

Instead of being a feared and fearsome event, then, mini-breakups revitalize our relationships. Even that nemesis, the other woman, can contribute to the sturdiness of our partnerships.

COLLEEN AND SERENA

In the seventies, Colleen and Serena came out together as novitiates. After they left the order, they took another set of vows: to stay together. For keeps. Twenty years later, they only shrug and smile knowingly when friends, eager to know the key to their enduring couplehood, inquire about their secret. Sometimes during these

grillings, Serena feels like an impostor. Over the years,
she has fallen in love with other women repeatedly. And
even though she has never acted on any of these
passions, she often wonders if her fantasies are
themselves a form of unfaithfulness.

Most of us have been taught that attractions for other
women constitute emotional betrayal. Sometimes these feelings and fantasies are so intense that we can't be sure if the
thoughts *are* deeds. Full of guilt and self-reproach, we tend
to suffer acutely from these perceived lapses in loyalty.

Yet within the breakup/reunion framework of intimacy,
virtual affairs are important—a form of leave-taking that
pushes us away from either/or thinking and toward more
complex togetherness. Yes, we love our long-term partners.
And, at the same time, we may be temporarily in lust with X
or Y. Nuanced and multiple truths mean roomier intimacies—love affairs with the tensile strength necessary to
thrive in the ambiguous and provisional worlds in which so
many of us now live.

The Breakup Within

Although attractions to outsiders are often the source of our
minibreakups, such attractions are not necessarily erotic.
Other acquaintances may be compelling for many reasons.
High powered or charismatic, they may stimulate us in
ways our mates cannot. And our partners may suffer by
comparison.

ARLIE, JAE, AND CHARLOTTE

They were the two most important women in her life: her mentor, Charlotte, the judge for whom she had clerked, and Jae, her new lover. Convinced that the two would hit it off famously, Arlie was elated that Charlotte and Jae would finally get to meet during a legal conference. But though the meeting happened, the anticipated bonding never materialized. Jae barely opened her mouth. She seemed small, awkward, even shabby next to the expansive and expensively coiffed Charlotte. Arlie felt embarrassed, ashamed. So dismayed, in fact, that for the first time since she had met Jae the year before, she had second thoughts about the relationship.

Certain ex-lovers or special friends, family members or admired co-workers seem to have the power to transform cherished intimates into irritating embarrassments. In the presence of a tight-lipped parent, for example, a lover's boyish charm will suddenly seem like a bad case of gender dysphoria, or her shyness irrefutable proof of her arrested development.

The feeling that we want to disown these impostors who claim to be our lovers is a common—and commonly denied—form of psychological breakup. When the episode is over and our feelings for our partners have returned to their previous loving status quo, this form of psychological revulsion tends to make us wonder if we are suffering from multiple personality disorder. But it is the relationships—not the partners—that are the multiples.

The Secret Breakup

Most relationships have a thousand expressions and moods—everything from abject disillusionment and discord to perfect serenity, from estrangement to soul blending. Such shifts can be baffling. But perhaps even harder to tolerate are the times when our relationships feel empty—so devoid of former feeling that they seem to be entirely lifeless.

YVONNE AND TIEG

> Yvonne and Tieg had been together for nine years. Both oldest daughters in large families, oncology nurses, and marathon runners, they had an extraordinary amount in common. But sometime during their fourth year together, their relationship began to feel flat. They wondered privately if this was what usually happened after the honeymoon intensity had dissipated or if something else, something more serious, was wrong. The "missing" feeling was strong enough to make each sure that even though they stayed together, and continued to enjoy the same things, in some mysterious unnamable way their original relationship had ended.

Rather than a fleeting emotional event like the breakup within, secret breakups are continuing, if intermittent, states of mind. At times the "missing" feeling may be so strong that partners wonder if they would be better off with someone else. At first glance, it might seem that such partners should take some action, *do* something about their irresolution. I'm not so sure.

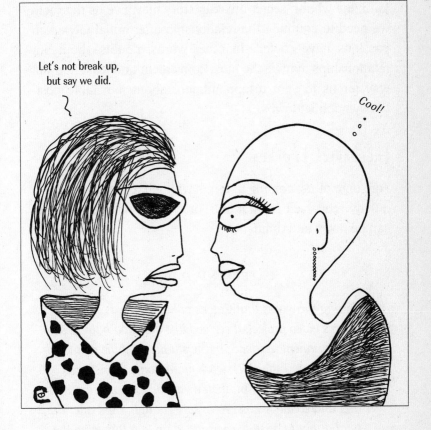

The lesbian reputation for passionate beginnings seems well deserved. Many of us who fall in love fall hard. After telling ourselves so emphatically that *this* is the one, we probably need a balancing story. Even if never spoken out loud, the what-if secret-breakup story may give us the room we need to continue the relationship after initial Olympian passions have cooled. In other words, doubts about our relationships may be the most convenient and least harmful way for us to vent disappointment about inevitable post-honeymoon letdowns.

The Basta! Breakup

For some of us, coming to terms with what *is* may require a quietly rehearsed separation. For others, such adjustments can be noisy and dramatic.

CATER AND DARIA

During the weeks that Cater's pal, Daria, was editing Cater's video project, it seemed like they had both taken up permanent residence in the studio. At some point during the round-the-clock work marathons, they started revising another script: their own story about being buddies and collaborators. And, sure enough, right after the final dubbing session, they ended up in a tangle on the sagging couch in back of the darkened room. The project's wrap segued perfectly into the beginning of an affair.

Though Cater was in an open relationship and could—and did—do pretty much what she wanted to, there were limits. And Daria wanted more than a date on Tuesday, a stolen interlude on Friday morning or Sunday afternoon when Sean, Cater's primary lover, was off playing golf or taking their dog to obedience class. So Daria and Cater fought, made love, and fought again. "This is it!" Daria would declare. "The end. Period. I can't get what I want from you. Or anybody else as long as I'm involved with you." And she would storm out.

After they hadn't seen each other for a few weeks, one or the other would think of a pretext: a book that had to be returned or a flyer about some upcoming event that the other should know about. And the cycle would start again. By the time their affair had hit the one-year mark, they had broken up, finally, irrevocably, on six separate occasions.

We all know it well—the endless breakup-reunion carousel: if we haven't gotten caught up ourselves, we know someone who has. Figuring out that a happy ending is impossible, we decide not to wait passively for an unhappy one. Instead, we pull the plug ourselves, pack up all our irreconcilable differences, and huff home. But a curious thing always seems to happen. Over time, the half-empty glass starts to look half-full. And when it comes to sex, that humble half-tumbler becomes an overflowing chalice. Just a little bit of contact, just enough to remind us of the problems, we tell ourselves. And soon we're back in for round umpteen.

Turbulent as it may seem, it is also predictable—even stable. Up and down, around and around. Perhaps the breakups last a little longer and the reunions get a little more intense. *Basta!* breakups are not anything any of us sign up for willingly. A bit melodramatic, they nevertheless expose the cadence in all relationships—and demonstrate our needs for both intimacy and autonomy. They also show us how very inventive we are at crafting and recrafting our love stories in ways that guarantee that our needs of the moment will be met.

The Intentional Breakup

Whatever their shape or form, we need our miniaturized endings. They soothe our anxiety about permanent separations and enrich the time we spend together. Microbreakups are so useful, in fact, that we may not want to wait for them to happen to us. We may choose to engineer our own.

TUP AND QUIN

Tup and Quin joked that as new freshmen, they fell in love during orientation week and immediately became disoriented. That was six years ago. Ever since then, they have been more or less inseparable. Until one day when Quin, picturing the next sixty years together, got itchy and worried that they were turning into merger queens. Tup, in turn, admitted that she had been having fantasies about what it might be like to date other women. It was true, they both had to admit. They had OD'd on togetherness. They needed some space and time apart. It turned out that their decision coincided with the plight of a friend who lived in another city. She needed a housesitter to take care of her dogs while she, in turn, became a live-in caretaker for a friend with AIDS. *Between jobs anyway, Tup volunteered.*

Before they went their separate ways, Tup and Quin hammered out the rules: During the two months they would spend apart, sex with other women was okay. But, they decided, pet names, overnights, and oral sex with anyone else was off-limits. Communication was trickier to figure out. Phone conversations might become an expensive habit—and, besides, they might turn into painful push-pull sessions. They settled on once-a-week snail mail contact: collages, poems, drawings, or letters—however the spirit moved them.

The sabbatical can be short or long, time-limited or open-ended. It can consist of a solitary stroll around the block or a month-long cross-country bike trip with a group of strangers. It may even be a standoff that looks and sounds like The End of the partnership. But don't let the masquerade fool you. The togetherness story is only dormant. The skirmish or disappointment or separation will be temporary. And the relationship will be stronger than ever.

Of course, there are permanent separations. And there are plenty of fights from hell—battles so draining and inconclusive that we wish we could extricate ourselves once and for all from partnerships that seem to be permanent power struggles.

No matter how hard we try, such chronic conflict may never be happily resolved. On the other hand, denial and suppression of the divisions between partners only rob us of the reunions that help us recognize the depth of our intimacy.

Naming and noticing microbreakups helps us recover from fear of breakups. Not only do we see that all breakups aren't bruisers, we also begin to tell new stories about temporary ruptures—funny anecdotes about the time we fell asleep on the couch or got a crush on that hot new coach. Telling such stories about the past makes such relationship time-outs normal, even comic events. Such storytelling also gives us both the practice and permission we need to craft the future.

Instead of dreading some cruel twist of fate that will wrench us away from our lovers, we can be in charge of how and when we come and go. Now we can tolerate separations; in fact, we can even plan them: everything from a solitary soak in the tub to a group pilgrimage to Lesbos. There are no limits to the separations we can devise. Why, instead of waiting until relationships end, we can even arrange to break up at the beginning.

The Get-Together Breakup, or I Married an Alien

The bruiser breakup story gets its power from the standard forever-after fable. If we hadn't been trained to think in terms of perfect matches that last a lifetime, relationship endings wouldn't feel like emotional Armageddons.

One way to deactivate forever-after is to start to tune in to and appreciate alternate love stories: those tales of short-term partnerships and niche love, of Net-amours and passionate friendships described in the previous chapter. But there is another remedy for the devastating domino effect caused by the forever-after story. What if we continued to tell the true-love tale . . . but with a slight twist? Instead of emphasizing seamless unity, what if our romances featured fractures and friction?

Most of us already have scraps of just such stories in our repertoires. And we use them as needed: "Of course she doesn't pick up after herself. She grew up with a nanny. In my family I *was* the nanny," or "Of course we don't agree about how much to save or spend. After all, I'm a Leo, and she's a Capricorn with Taurus rising. Aaaarrrgh!"

Such fragmentary explanations bridge the gulfs that periodically divide partners. But what if the framework for the whole relationship consisted of a permanent chasm—a division so profound that togetherness could be achieved only through a continuous series of delicate, brilliant bridging maneuvers? In such a framework, differences, divisions, perhaps even misunderstandings, would seem natural and normal, and togetherness a somewhat disorientating, if delicious, interlude. How might we craft such a story?

Capricorn and Leo point us in the right narrative direction. But in order to spin the kind of yarn we need, we may have to venture far beyond our celestial suburbs—to zip beyond Orion and the Big Dipper, beyond the goat and the lion, to a very distant galaxy.

Instead of a being part of a perfect mirror match between two queer Homo sapiens, let's say that by some quirk of fate we have fallen in love with an alien, a creature from

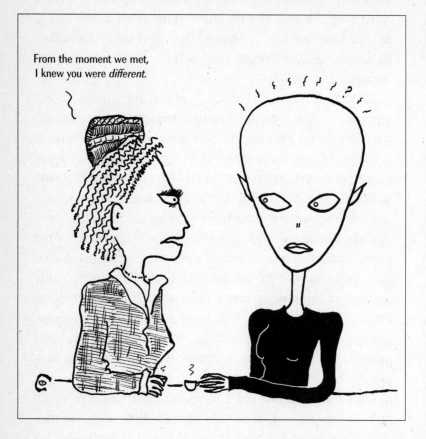

Xega 4. She fools us at first, but her earthling masquerade soon becomes transparent. The habits chalked up at first to eccentricity are really just a reflection of her faraway culture. It comes as a shock, but the alien is an utterly enchanting creature. So, in the interests of interplanetary diversity, we decide to make the best of it.

The scenario isn't so far-fetched. After all, most of us, at one time or another, have successfully coexisted with aliens. Take cats, for example. Our culinary and toilet habits are quite different from those of our feline companions, yet we don't begrudge them theirs. In fact, out of respect for the differences, we may even buy them catnip and kitty litter. Ditto for different generations of our own species. We wouldn't be caught dead wearing the same clothes or sporting the same hairstyles as our parents or kids. Yet even though we can't grasp why older and younger generations favor particular hair hues, we don't hesitate to compliment them on their blue dos.

When it comes to the majority of those near and dear to us, we tell the alien story effortlessly, without even thinking about it. Yet our bemused tolerance of eccentricity dead-ends when it comes to our mates. We are hurt and puzzled, or angry and frustrated, for example, when partners won't pick up piles of paper or clothes or when they forget to do their half of the chores.

But what if we already had the alien story in place? Then, as soon as we realize our wrongheaded partner is not an Earthling, we will assume her quirks are part of her Xegan heritage. Perhaps she hails from a z-gravity galaxy. In such a free-floating atmosphere, objects tend to hover rather than

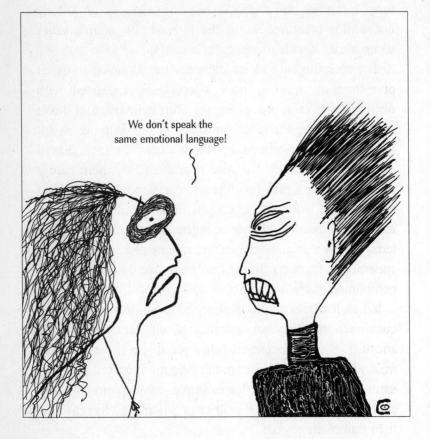

be placed. Consequently, the elevation of piles of clothes or papers, which is offensive to those with an earthbound sense of order, is *comme il faut* to the Xegans. In fact, back on planet Earth, piles are the perfect remedies for Xegan homesickness. Or perhaps the fifty-fifty division of chores, so prized on terra firma, seems to the prescient denizens of Xega a foolish fiction, a denial of the far more complex web of give-and-take interactions they are tuned in to. We wouldn't want our favorite Xegan to forsake her ways any more than we would expect a cat to enjoy soaking in a hot bath.

The lovers-as-aliens story isn't entirely fabricated. Often our lesbian partners come from different classes or ethnic backgrounds. They speak different emotional languages. And their sexual habits, domestic customs, and sleep patterns certainly suggest that they belong to a different species. In short, they may as well have come from different galaxies.

If we tell the I-Married-an-Alien story, we will anticipate quirkiness and misunderstandings. Instead of assuming we and our partners will blend into a seamless whole, we would expect plenty of microbreakups (she sleeps on Saturday morning while I jog; the kitchen is my turf; the living room, hers).

In time, Xegans and Earthlings can come to understand, and even appreciate, each other's ways. There have even been reports that, with enough exposure, a few Xegans and Earthlings have actually become bicultural.

Cultivating the Art of the Microbreakup

The bruiser breakup is a story that those of us who have "been there, done that" can tell in gory detail. It is an instructive tale of death and rebirth, a dyke passage as important as falling in love or coming out. Valuable as it is, however, it isn't the only breakup story. Unfortunately, though, the more it is told, the more it will drown out the other more subtle stories we might tell about loss and separation.

We know dozens of ways to express love to our partners. We cuddle or chat, leave notes or bring home treats. With each of these gestures, we tell our partners a different story about caring. We need to be able to tell just as many stories about disappointments and interruptions, standoffs and microbreakups. We need stories about getting in each other's hair and sleeping apart, about evenings out with friends and attractions to other women. And we need to practice these time-outs from intimacy as automatically as we might offer to rub a partner's neck after a hard day at work.

We need to know dozens of stories about the going part of the coming and going that comprises intimacy. Such a supply of tales, tapped daily, shows us that each breakup isn't going to turn into the Big One. And, eventually, such little stories will add up to much more lively relationships.

As long as we allow breakup terror to shape all our tomorrows, our own ability to storytell whatever future we want will be sadly limited. We will find ourselves dotting the *i*'s and crossing the *t*'s of our new love stories before we have even met our partners-to-be. Because of our anxiety, we dare not even ask ourselves the question that is at the heart of every good love story: what happens next? We are terrified that we *know* what might happen next. But this eagerness to avoid catastrophe doesn't keep us safe. It only robs our love stories of suspense, mystery, and romance.

Chapter 4

Love and Sex, Plural

Despite its apparent timelessness, the story of a lesbian partnership based on true love is really a newfangled invention. Of course, women have always fallen in love with each other. But regardless of whether their amores blossomed in medieval convents or Restoration drawing rooms, Victorian brothels or fin de siècle boarding schools, chances are passions between women were limited, confined to stolen moments in secret alcoves or notes passed hurriedly in the dark. Much as we might want to claim these clandestine lovers as the foremothers of today's lesbian couples, we can't. Sad to say, these branches of the family tree withered away in secrecy and silence far too often to have had much influence on contemporary dyke love.

If today's lesbian couples have anyone to thank (or curse) for their faith in the triumph of true love, it is heterosexuals. Not the traditional, settle-down-and-get-married straight couples. Our real spiritual foremothers and forefathers are the Guineveres and Lancelots, the highborn ladies and the lowly knights who, despite their passionate devotion, could never hope to be joined in holy matrimony.

For most of recorded history, marriage has been a practical arrangement—an efficient way to produce a plentiful supply of help around the house and garden. The formation of an in-law alliance with a potentially hostile neighbor never hurt, either. But even for hets, tying this obviously beneficial knot hasn't always been easy. For one thing, traditionally, brides have been big-ticket items. As a result, suitors without property or prospects were simply out of luck.

Too far down on the rungs of the sibling ladder to inherit anything more than a good name and a suit of armor, the knights of medieval Europe put the best possible spin on their leftover status. They proclaimed their passions for the remote and lovely ladies already married off to luckier, land-rich suitors. The sublime sentiments expressed in the poetry and love songs of these Galahads-come-lately started a new romantic trend. The idealization of one's beloved became as indispensable to love as contracts were to marriage.

Centuries had to pass, and plenty of royal heads had to roll, before the two very separate tracks of love and marriage began to converge. Before the new American colonies declared their independence from England in 1775, for example, only one out of four colonial magazines credited romantic love as a solid basis for marriage. Shortly after the

American Revolution, however, love's approval ratings shot up. References to prenuptial romance in popular periodicals tripled. Not only was love in the air, it had also taken its place among the inalienable rights of each and every citizen of the fledgling democracies.

The rest, as they say, is herstory. In fact, that proverbial horse and carriage, love and marriage, is now almost within hailing distance of lesbian couples. The legal recognition of our partnerships will finally bring the painfully slow evolution of lesbian couplehood to a close. Or will it? A butch bragging session at a party I attended recently suggests that our couples stories are still undergoing major revisions.

Love, Plural

The party was supposed to be a surprise. As the twenty guests huddled together in a back bedroom trying to pass the time before the birthday girl arrived, somebody proposed that we make a collective tally of the dyke years we had logged. As each of us stage-whispered our numbers—our current age minus the number of our pre-coming-out years—a self-appointed secretary jotted down the figures. She chewed her pencil thoughtfully as she looked over the numbers and then announced that she was deducting thirty years for patent lies. (For example, insistent that she had been a dyke in utero, one woman in the room claimed to have come out at birth.) Finally, pausing for effect, the secretary announced the grand total came to 389 queer-years. Her announcement provoked a round of approving aha's and muted applause. Not that we were surprised. Most of us were in our thirties or forties and had been out for decades. Still, the collective wisdom represented by such a sum deserved acknowledgment.

When the phone rang, we all jumped. It was the birthday girl's lover, sneaking a quick call from a gas station en route. They were caught in a traffic jam.

Someone commandeered a bottle of champagne from the kitchen. Another of the guests broke open the box of naked lady truffles she had brought. Our tally keeper proposed another round of impromptu research. This time, she suggested that each guest scribble on a scrap of paper her lifetime total of women lovers. In order to prevent the "research" from degenerating into an alpha-butch contest, the survey was to be conducted anonymously. Each woman scribbled her stats on a scrap of paper, wadded it up, and tossed it into the secretary's cap. With a flourish, she drew out each wad, unfolded it, and jotted down its secret contents. After another bout of concentrated pencil chewing, she announced that, collectively, the group could boast 241 lovers. There was another round of applause, and someone joked that the number probably represented a total of six women, in different combinations with each other. Someone else quipped that most of them were sitting right there in the room. After this observation, our tally taker opened the Korbel and started pouring. And everyone else started talking.

Mostly, the group was composed of pros, veterans of dozens of domestic war and peace times. When these women started to tell all, even the shortest buzz cuts in the group had plenty of hair to let down. Most had begun their dyke careers as believers in forever-after, and each, in her own way, was still a romantic. But over time they had fine-tuned their all-time favorite love story. For some women, Eros—albeit a modified form—still played the lead. Others had replaced romantic love with a more comfortable, long-haul brand of commitment. Still others, after years of trial and error, had come up with new hybrids. By the time we uncorked the second bottle of champagne, the group was in the middle of conducting yet another unofficial survey. This time around, we began musing about the key to lasting love and durable relationships. Here are some of our tried-and-true formulas.

Bifocal Love

Each of the coupled lesbians was already an old hand at love when she had gotten together with her current partner. The magic soul lightning had struck not only twice but dozens of times in the same place. In fact, each woman had become so familiar with the trancelike aspects of passion that she had developed her own inner adviser. At the first suggestion of a new romance, the sardonic voice of this commentator could be detected above the loudest sighs and moans: "Well, here we are again. Feels as good now as it did the last forty times." Or "Yes, she is absolutely charming . . ." then a pregnant pause, ". . . for now."

It was as though these sexual sages had acquired a set of bifocals through which they regarded both new and more seasoned passions. There was in-love and there was long-love; love-lite and megaton love; perishable love and cher-ishable love. These two-tiered versions had been very functional. They had allowed the couples to revere romance at the same time as they restricted it. Since passion was being simultaneously honored and humored, fresh outbreaks of Eros were much less likely to ruffle these women's long-term relationships.

Collaborative Love

Everyone agreed that Eros was exquisite, a not-to-be-missed experience. But several of the guests had chosen to base their relationships on entirely different passions. All the energy of one couple, for example, had been funneled into their new baby.

In addition to their regular jobs, another couple had chosen to moonlight. Every dime they earned was being squirreled away for the country land they hoped to buy one day.

Most of us harbor secret dreams. Perhaps one day we will travel to the Serengeti or open our own lesbian-only bed-and-breakfast or mount a campaign that will preserve a pristine forest. And, on the rare occasions when we let our intimates in on our private plans, we often regret it. Perhaps they are skeptical, or, even worse, their feigned enthusiasm is transparent. We know perfectly well what they are *really* thinking. Yet, just imagine how it might feel to have one's private passion wholeheartedly shared by a mate.

To most of us, dream lovers are mirages—imaginings too good to be true. But for certain couples such ideal partners are not at all far-fetched. They are simply collaborators who share our zeal for a particular enterprise. Instead of scoffing at our visions, these special lovers codream our dreams with us.

According to the dream team lovers among the guests, collaborating on beloved projects generated a higher togetherness quotient than falling in love ever had. In fact, these alternative passions had proven so compelling to these couples that the old head-over-heels brand of love seemed almost quaint—as dusty and denuded as Xanadu.

Eighty-Percent Love

One of the partygoers announced that in the old days she would have left a lover who met only eighty percent of her needs. Now, merely twenty percent short of a perfect score was a good reason to stay with her partner. Not to mention that after a while, she had even become attached to her lover's shortcomings.

Another woman said that she no longer thought in terms of forever-after. She would be delighted if she could achieve her five-year plan.

Romantic love and idealization are so closely entwined that it is hard to conceive of one without the other. And in fact, when we realize that the grouch incapable of a civil grunt before her morning coffee is not the dream lover we once swooned over, romance takes a dive. At this juncture, some partners quietly mourn the end of the honeymoon; others try to rekindle the old passion or, failing that, hunt for a new heartthrob. Still others begin to practice the art of good-enough love. While not exactly cherishing their partner's morning grumps or evening couch-potato tendencies, these long-termers tend to regard their mates' foibles with amusement and affection.

A certain fondness for a partner's quirks hardly qualifies as earth-moving passion. On the other hand, eighty-percent love, in its own small way, can be more ideal and idealizing than the kind that makes the love meter soar. After all, it is easy in the beginning—when we hardly know our mate—to marvel at her every word and gesture. It is even more of a marvel, however, to feel some of the same glow even after we have taken off the rose-colored glasses.

Accelerated Love

One guest said she gone to great lengths to cure herself of what a long string of exes had told her was her sex addiction. After going to plenty of Sex and Love Addicts Anonymous meetings, she realized that she was in the wrong place. She wasn't an addict or, for that matter, even sexually obsessed. She simply fell in love quickly and easily.

"Real" love is supposed to be a magical event, something that occurs so rarely that we are obliged to take it seriously. But when quantity is added to the usual scarce helpings of love, the meaning of the experience also changes.

For romance adepts, love is simply a natural, delightful, and effortless part of getting to know someone. Many some-ones. It is not the basis of a permanent partnership. Long-term relationships, which often come with exclusive commit-ments, may not suit the easy-access group. Instead of relying on one partner, their needs for continuity and emotional contact may be met by friends or by several concurrent lovers.

On the other hand, such low-threshold love does not automatically preclude long-term partnerships. If both partners specialize in easy-access eros, they will find it much easier to craft rules that allow for each other's proclivities. Mutual agreements about multiple lovers can make relationships betrayal-proof. And, when infidelity can be converted into official nonmonogamy, romance adepts frequently prove themselves to be loyal and durable mates.

Lesbians aren't the first to identify more than one variety of love. The Greeks, for all their misogynist ways (think of all those raped and pillaged goddesses), managed to come up with six types:

1. Obsessive love was characterized by agitation, sleeplessness, loss of appetite, and, if unreciprocated, heartache.
2. Altruistic love, in contrast, was patient and kind and never demanded reciprocity.
3. Playful love was fun.
4. Companionate love appeared after years of mutual contentment.
5. Realistic love, based on shared interests and backgrounds, culminated in sturdy, common-sense matches.
6. Eros, the love of beauty, was based on intense physical attraction. Erotic love, according to the Greeks, burned fiercely and died quickly.

Eros was much in evidence in the stories of the party guests. And their relationships had also blended playfulness and companionability, practicality and altruism. Besides displaying all the varieties of love familiar in Sappho's day, the partygoers had come up with a few postmodern sequels to the old love story. These new versions had evolved gradually over time—so slowly that the bifocalists and the collaborators, the eighty-percenters and the fast-forward lovers hadn't even realized how far they had diverged from forever-after. If the truth-or-dare spirit of the party hadn't prevailed, these alternative styles might have remained unnamed and unnoticed. As it turned out, the group displayed even more storytelling talent when it came to sex.

Sex, Plural

When the birthday girl finally arrived, she was duly serenaded by the throng of well wishers. Still dazed, she was ushered to her pile of booty. When the first gift, a python-sized double dildo, snaked out of its wrapping, I realized the whoppers had only just begun. The tales had shifted, however. Instead of hearing about past loves, now we were in for a multimedia show-and-tell about future sex.

Next came a transparent teddy. Then, in quick succession, she unwrapped a butch/femme etiquette book, some fur-lined handcuffs, and a lifetime supply of prelubed latex gloves. Quite a change from the haul of labyris earrings, women's Muzak tapes, and Amazon gewgaws the new forty-year-old had probably received on the occasion of her thirtieth birthday.

FIN-DE-SIÈCLE
SAPPHIC SEX PRACTICES

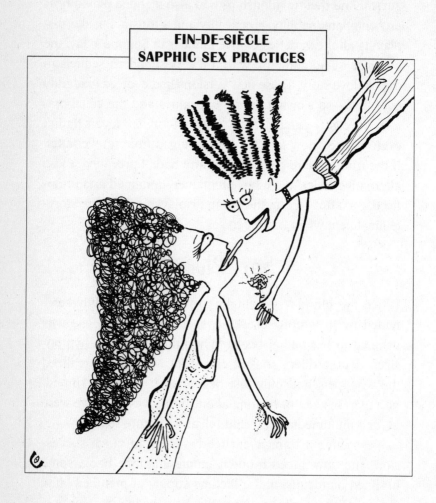

When it comes to the varieties of love, the partygoers could have taught Sappho a thing or two. And the authors of the Kama Sutra might have added an instructive chapter or two to their opus if they had they been privy to the radical sex practices of these *fin-de-siècle* Sapphists.

(K)nights in Black Leather

The medieval knights were social misfits. They were also pied pipers of romance. Perhaps it has taken a group just as marginal, a new breed of ragtag warriors, to point us in another direction. The sexual proclivities of sadists and masochists, gender-benders and polymorphous perverts, prostitutes and performance artists may horrify the squeamish and seem heretical to feminists. Nevertheless, this motley brigade has expanded the range of stories all lesbians can tell. Sex renegades have shown us that sex need not be passion sex or even relationship sex. The intrepid band of erotic innovators has even managed to separate sex from the pleasures most of us assume are part and parcel of "doing it."

It hasn't been an easy task. Most maverick storytellers learn a code as rigorous as anything practiced by the knights in King Arthur's court. To tell against-the-grain stories takes training, discipline, and perseverance. In fact, the whips and restraints that are *de rigueur* in s/m scenes may have a dual purpose. Besides keeping bottoms in their place, perhaps such an arsenal is necessary to keep the ubiquitous romantic story at bay.

Even though exotic erotica will never replace romantic vanilla, the trickle-down effect of these new sexual stories is evident everywhere: in the mound of toys accumulating next to the birthday girl; in workshop bulletins and classified ads; even in my day-to-day exchanges with friends.

Not long ago, an old chum called to tell me about her latest setback. She had been girlfriend hunting without much success. One evening, she said, she felt the old familiar surge toward a woman she worked with on the staff of a gay newspaper. Feeling certain that her interest was reciprocated, my friend proposed that the two of them get together after work sometime. The response: "You know I'm into s/m" (a detail my friend had conveniently overlooked). "I only get together with people I can play with. Sorry. And I know you too well, anyway."

Weeks after the rejection, my friend was still trying to make sense of such topsy-turvy mating rituals.

My own introduction to the changing dykegeist was less jarring. A few years ago I went to see a performance by Annie Sprinkle, self-proclaimed-porn-star-turned-sacred-temple-prostitute. As Annie started to vibrate to orgasm onstage in concert with a handful of her Sapphic sisters, the audience was given rattles and encouraged to participate in the mounting rhythm. Never a fan of any organized religion before, I found myself an instant convert to this brand of evangelesbianism. A woman in the row behind me must have sensed my enthusiasm. During the postorgasmic glow of intermission, she leaned over and asked me slyly if it had been as good for me as it had been for her.

Fortunately, sex has always been amazingly accommodating. A Rorschach rich enough to encompass whatever anybody wants to read into it, sex has been proof of salvation or sin, source of pleasure or pain, freely given or forcefully extorted. Even within the boundaries of Lesbian Nation, it is being constantly tugged and tweaked into new shapes.

In the past few years, dozens of new stories about arousal, fantasy, and performance have escaped from the romantic love-sex net. So much so that lately it is not the unenlightened het hordes but dykes themselves who want to know what we *do* in bed. What exactly *is* the lesbian common denominator? Orgasms? Hardly. Two partners? Not necessarily. Physical touch? Online dykes disagree. Even female partners are optional for some lesbians. But what if we stopped even trying to connect all the dots? Stopped trying to jam relaxation and arousal, lust and love, familiarity and surprise, calculation and spontaneity into a single event?

If we let sex relax, it falls quite naturally into separate activities. To be sure, the new divisions may be fuzzy around the edges, and there is bound to be plenty of overlap. Even so, each of the new sections has a different purpose. Each can be a vehicle for different aspects of ourselves.

The Sex Menu

If we pluralize sex—promote it from an "it" to a multiple—passion sex is still an option. But now, it is one of several choices on the menu. Take your pick. Or if nothing proves appealing, make up your own menu.

Maintenance Sex

Predictable sex. Yuck. Bor-r-ring. Considered next to the rush of passion, maintenance sex *is* less than electrifying. But what if we take another look at what so many of us are already doing? If we view maintenance sex as an activity that is completely independent of—separate from—passion sex, then we are free to consider it in its own right. Thus named and noticed, a onetime boring habit can be upgraded into a sweet acknowledgment, a certification of togetherness.

Orgasmic habits make no starburst claims. More ritual than genital, they are simply small, frequent valentines. And just as once a year we might hunt for just the right card to commemorate February 14, once a week or so we find the right moment to celebrate our partnerships with an orgasm or two.

HOLLIS AND JESSICA

Hollis and Jessica have their orgasms down to a finely tuned art. Hollis does Jessica first, then obligingly flips over on her back so Jessica can do her. Sometimes they even compete to see who can come the fastest. They do it once a week, rain or shine, whether or not they feel like it. Sometimes Hollis would prefer gardening, or Jessica hates tearing herself away from her mystery. But afterward, when they feel closer, they're always glad they have taken the time.

Because partners who practice orgasmic rituals can't predict that they will be at all inclined to touch or be touched at 10:00 A.M. every Saturday, they rely on certain techniques to awaken slumbering libidos. Some women claim that their vibrators sustain them. Still others tune in to unspoken, unshared fantasies when their partners stimulate them. Others have asymmetrical orgasms: one partner comes and one doesn't.

Orgasms have great potential to be naturally occurring rituals. In the first place, rituals should be performed with some regularity. Since orgasms tend to be habit forming, they seem to satisfy the criterion effortlessly.

Second, rituals are special events. Our genitals are private. Only special people get to touch them. Ergo, our lovers are special.

Third, rituals are clearly cordoned off from the rest of life's activities. So are orgasms. Some lesbians report that they can come while driving, but such activities belong in the derring-do-me category of sex rather than the maintenance ritual sextion.

Finally, it's important to know how to end rituals. In the case of orgasms, we can count on our bodies to tell us when the ritual is over.

A couple I met in a Net chatroom reported an interesting variation on the genital-touching ritual. In their case, the genitals in question belonged to lovers outside the relationship. Before either partner planned an encounter with someone else, she made a special point of asking her primary lover for permission. Consulted in this way, the partner never exercised her veto power. The couple called it their Mother-May-I ritual and attributed their longevity as a couple to its regular performance.

What is significant about such rituals is not the touching of genitals, but rather that partners have worked out familiar, synchronized routines, stylized dances by which they mark off a special space that includes just the two of them.

Rituals are the way we perform our relationships. They are miniaturized commitment ceremonies. Less flashy, they are nonetheless just as sustaining as more choreographed big bashes.

Scene Sex

Maintenance sex is one type of sex that is distinct from passion sex. Another distinct category is scene sex. Improvised erotic theatricals have nothing to do with maintenance or passion. In fact, these psychodramas have very little to do with our present-day partners.

BUNNY RUTH AND TULSA

Early in their relationship, Bunny Ruth and Tulsa became addicts. It all began when they wandered into a Goodwill store to kill time before a movie. They emerged so loaded down with their new purchases that they decided to skip the movie—to go home and make their own. It was the beginning of many such shopping excursions.

When their booty of thirdhand uniforms, army surplus boots, frayed silk pj's, oversized suits and skinny ties, slinky negligees, sling-back mules, and bridal gowns started spilling out of their closet, they built a second one just for their customized collection.

When the spirit moved them, they would shuffle through their wardrobe, select a few items, and begin to improvise a scene. Their private theatricals usually followed a predictable plotline: one of them was going about her business (anything from delivering pizzas to getting married) when she was derailed—seduced, coerced, or cajoled by some unexpected intruder into doing something naughty and totally inappropriate.

Given half a chance, most of us will tell a very private tale—divulge a private enchantment we may not even know is lurking inside of us. Add a few props, encouragement from a witness who can be trusted, and the tales turn tawdry. Old secrets tumble out. Ancient wrongs are revealed and righted.

Oddly enough, the best revenge for the old violations of our bodies or spirits is a fantasy replay of the original dirty deed. With one slight change. In the new version, the one-time victim turns the tables on the perpetrator by having a better time than her oppressor ever did.

Sex therapist and researcher Jack Morin surveyed more than 350 people of all races, classes, and sexual orientations about their turn-ons. From his interviews, he concluded that many of us have learned to transform unfinished emotional business from childhood and adolescence into sexual scripts. An old parent-child power imbalance, for example, can be transformed into a sexual fantasy in which one anonymous intruder forces sex upon an unwilling victim. By choreographing the scene in her head and by moving back and forth between the two roles, the fantasizer can safely express aggression toward a parent, undo some of the powerlessness she felt as a child, and absolve herself of any guilt about incestuous feelings. Besides being both arousing and healing, such core scenes lend themselves to endless variations.

With the help of a wig or a waggish dildo, we can be our worst nightmares *and* our best fantasies. We need not confine our temporary biodiversity to erotic stunts. One couple I worked with used animal hand puppets to fight their battles. Once they assumed their alternative personae as Mrs. Jaws and T. Rex, respectively, they growled and roared, munched and crunched on each other until their animus was discharged. They would never have acted in such beastly fashion in street clothes or, for that matter, in their birthday suits.

Couples may even want to take their playlets on the road. An easy warm-up is going out in public with just one piece of playful plumage—perhaps a jockstrap concealed under jeans or a single strand of dime-store pearls draped over a T-shirt. Simply sporting a token of the beauty or beast within can transform dates, or even trips to the grocery store, into riveting psychodramas. Oscar Wilde observed that we are least candid when we are "ourselves." Give us masks, he advised, and we will tell the truth.

Passion Sex

As soon as we separate maintenance sex and scene sex from the perturbations of passion sex, we can begin to notice and appreciate their piquant flavors and functions. By the same token, once we liberate passion sex from the hot-cold sex continuum, we can gain new insights about the form and function of the magic meltdown.

THE LOVERS

They couldn't get enough of each other. When they got close enough to touch, they could almost see blue light crackling between them, could almost hear the sssszzzt of an electrical charge. Perhaps as a way of paying its respects to their otherworldly state, time stopped. Eating and sleeping also became irrelevant, quaint activities pursued by ordinary people.

Psychologist and author Dorothy Tennov coined the word *limerence* to describe the altered states reported so frequently by new lovers. After interviewing five hundred people of all sexual persuasions about their experiences, she came up with a list of limerent attributes. Those in love, she found, tended to idealize and focus exclusively on the beloved. Other people and concerns quickly faded into the background. Obstacles in the form of misunderstandings, family disapproval, and even outright rejections seemed only to heighten limerence.

In his book *The Homosexual Matrix*, psychologist C. A. Trip echoed some of the same themes. Love, he concluded, thrived on adversity: "Impediments of some kind (accidental or deliberate) are *necessary* precursors in the psychology of sexual arousal," he wrote. The need for such obstacles, he goes on to say, is even evident in the push-pull sexual dance of certain one-celled organisms.

Still other theorists maintain that the in-love feeling is generated by phenylethylamine (PEA)—an amphetaminelike substance produced by the brain's pleasure centers. Bolstering the neurochemical theory is the frequency with which such euphoric states are reported by those *not* in love. The fact that ecstasy can be triggered by widely different activities—everything from mountain climbing to contemplating one's newborn—suggests that the potential for intense pleasure resides in most of us. Both euphoria triggers and thresholds, however, seem to vary dramatically from person to person.

Despite differences in perspectives, all these theories about bliss share something: each in its own way provides us with a story that runs counter to the once-in-a-lifetime, one-and-only stories we tell ourselves when we are in love. In other words, ecstasy explanations—whether chemical or psychological—supply the bifocals that the love-worn dykes at the surprise party had accumulated through experience.

No matter how we acquire them, these bifocals are important. They allow us to enjoy limerence, even while we can see around the edges of its eternal promises.

Ex Sex

On the new sex menu, one brand of the old "it" still remains. Though a current choice, "it" depends on a retrospective view of what has already happened. Ex sex, the residue of sex past, is the special bond that exists between ex-lovers.

AFTER FOREVER-AFTER

They hadn't seen each other, even talked, for years. It didn't matter. It turned out that they were so habituated to each other's way of thinking, of moving, that they resumed their old intimacy effortlessly. They caught up on each other's news and, as the day wore on, speculated about their ability to be instantly close when, in the interval between get-togethers, so much had happened. They didn't feel as comfortable with other friends or even with current lovers. Eventually they decided it was because they had once been lovers, had known each other's bodies inside and out. The afterglow of that connection, they decided, accounted for the magical bond they shared with no one else.

It's hard to pinpoint the quality so often shared by one-time sexual partners. Ex sex is an ease, a special comfort—both a security that cannot be ruffled and a closeness that cannot be interrupted by time or space. Ex sex is also the glue that often binds many of our unconventional families together. One newly (and frequently) unpartnered friend of mine tells me—only half in jest—that she is no longer sure if she should start dating or merely begin to "interview" new women to see if, sometime in the future, they have the potential to become part of her family of ex-lovers.

Ex sex may or may not include genital contact. But even on the occasions when it does, ex-lovers are engaged with each other in a distinctly different way from partners who have maintenance or scene or passion sex. They are tapping into an underground store of old memories, an auld lang syne of intimacy. They are having ex sex.

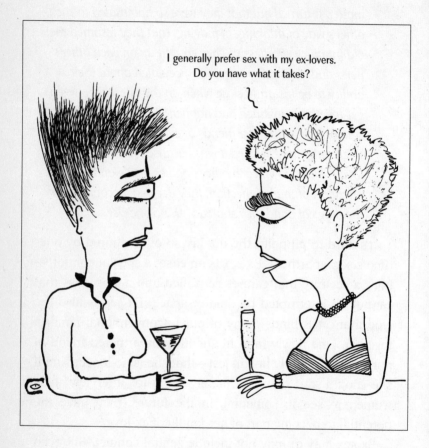

Parenthetically, current partners need not break up to enjoy the blessings of ex sex. They need only declare themselves ex-lovers. This simple announcement might do more to end lesbian bed death than all the workshops, sex toys, and exotic vacations in the world.

Maintenance and scene sex, passionate and ex sex are only a few of the possible choices. Scroll down the menu a little farther, and you will find still other options: there are spanking-the-mouse cyber encounters; the devouring sex hunger of lovers who know they will be separated; the genital incidentalism of old friends stranded in a cabin during a snowstorm; and the tentative puppy piles of dorm mates intent on having an orgiastic tale to tell the day after.

Each of these sexualities (as well as the dozens of others we might conjure up) has a different purpose, stirs different feelings, and follows (or breaks) different rules. Within sex plural there is room for these activities and dozens of others not yet named or even imagined.

Creating Our Own Menus

Because we've all been brainwashed by the single-event sex story, most of us don't even know that we are longtime practitioners of sex plural. Yet, chances are we've conducted our own private rituals and starred in our own guerrilla theater pieces. Few of us have escaped spells of ex sex or passion sex. Once we become conscious of our separate stories, we will be free to embellish them and tell yet more tales.

The tyranny of the single-sex story becomes more vivid if we shift, for just a moment, to an entirely different context. Picture, for a minute, the long parade of official questionnaires you have filled out in your life. Now, imagine how you might feel, if coming upon the section that asks for your age or your ethnicity, you find only one possible choice. There is a box labeled "Eighteen years old," but no place to check if you happen to be under or over the voting age. Or, say, there is only one ethnic box labeled Asian American. If you happen to be Hispanic or African American or of European descent, you look in vain for some other boxes. Failing to find them, you might be perplexed or miffed at such an obvious misprint. Somehow, somewhere, you would probably find a way to insert your own identifying information.

A single yes/no sex story is even more ludicrous than a one-box questionnaire. At least there are twenty-one-year-old Asian Americans who *could* check the correct box on the form. But one-size-sex fits absolutely no one.

Passion will always be precious. Equally precious are the many versions of sex and love told by experienced storytellers. As soon as we don our bifocals, we realize that the real magic—the ability to endow an adored lover with magic or to create relationships that really matter—resides in each of us.

Thanks to our enhanced vision and our multiple versions, love no longer needs to be a precipitous plunge into forever-after. Instead, it can be any one of several delightful flights that, depending on conditions, we can cancel or continue. The choice is ours.

Chapter 5

Sophie's (or Annie's or Sue's or Diana's) Choice: Passion or Permanence?

"What am I going to do?" Sophie looks at me imploringly. "I just know I'm going to do something I will regret. This drop-dead gorgeous dyke has joined the symphony. Black curly hair. Olive skin. The whole bit." Sophie hesitates, swallows hard, and continues. "Her name is Marta, and she plays the cello like an angel. She sits right next to me. We've started going out for lattes after rehearsals. You've got to help me."

Even though Sophie is a new client, I have heard this heartbreaker before. It is a story told haltingly, in fits and starts, by anguished lesbians who come to therapy alone. Their partners, they tell me, are still in the dark about what is going on. The timing couldn't be worse. They have just bought a house or had a baby or planned a commitment ceremony together. And now there is someone new. Perhaps she is a co-worker, a new friend, or the guide on a recent business trip to Europe—a polyglot who, besides being fluent in five languages, is able to decode the secret languages of souls.

Sophie ticks off her options as though she were juggling hot coals: perhaps she should confess the infatuation and throw herself on her lover's mercy; or she should just keep her mouth shut and try to raise the lust quotient at home; or perhaps she should she go for it: a scorched-earth policy. Propose an elopement to the new flame . . . or at least a torrid afternoon.

Sophie gnaws her nails. "Of course you can't tell me what to do," she laughs nervously. "But I hope you will."

It is a dilemma that cries out for resolution. Preserve an old relationship or pursue a new one? Which shall it be? Permanence or passion? Cherished intimate or new fling? With Sophie's long-term relationship hanging in the balance, the suspense is contagious. All pretense of therapeutic sangfroid dropped, I, too, perch anxiously on the edge of my chair.

But wait. Why such urgency? What's the hurry?

During the "emergency session" with Sophie, it takes me a while to realize that we are both being stampeded by the togetherness story. It has decreed that we must choose, on the spot, whom to hunker down with for eternity or at least whom to spend the night with—whom to include, whom to exclude. But if we refuse to go along with the familiar either/or plot and resist tidying up an admittedly ambiguous situation, we have a chance to craft a fresh story. In fact, all the elements of a good mystery are already present.

Sophie is indeed mystified. Practically overnight she has been transformed from a loving partner to . . . what? She isn't sure. All she knows is that everything is strange. In the presence of the new cellist, ordinary gestures, glances, hesitations, even casual remarks have become exotic flashes. The air is heavy, almost palpable. Colors vibrate with an odd intensity, and ears buzz with the soft purr of not-quite-decipherable sounds.

It is a twilight zone that deserves more exploration. But how to stall, to wait? How to allow the loose ends to simply dangle? What if we apply the tricks of the trade used by the master storyteller?

The Art of the Sequel

Long after first falling under his spell, I found out that at one time Dickens's cliffhangers had been serialized, a nineteenth-century *As the World Turns*. His talent, like the soap opera writers of today, resided in his ability to defer endings. Dickens's muse was necessity. His never-ending stories had to keep pace with the needs of his ever-expanding brood of offspring. Yet another hairpin turn, another shocking revelation in his epic tales meant another leg of mutton, another month of lodging paid for.

Dickens was the master of sequels. We, too, can practice the art of sustained mystery and adventure. There is a simple first step: instead of immediately labeling new intimates as either friends or lovers, we can linger in the unmapped regions in between such definitions.

Sophie shifts uncomfortably from one side of her chair to the other, trying, it seems, to wriggle off the horns of her dilemma.

"How about not doing anything?" I suggest. "Just see what happens?"

Sophie gives me an incredulous look. "But I've got to do something. I can't go on like this."

"Okay. Let's just try a short experiment. Just go out with Marta after another rehearsal . . . maybe two. But this time don't pressure yourself. Just see what it is like to be with her without having to decide anything."

As it turned out, Sophie was lucky. She came back to tell me that Marta had gotten involved with her downstairs neighbor. "Whew, close call," was Sophie's only comment. But she didn't call off their postrehearsal get-togethers. Now that Marta was involved elsewhere, the adventure wasn't quite as nerve-racking. She could even savor the irresolution—the what-ifs and maybes.

A few months later, Sophie came in to report that Marta had broken up with the downstairs dyke and was "available" again. The urge to "do something" had come up again. But this time around, the impulse had been only a weak echo of Sophie's original desire. And anyway, she was really enjoying her relationship with Marta in its current form. The strangely exciting buzz had never gone away.

Delicious as the feelings were, they were also subtle. Sophie was sure that they would never survive the rush of hot, new sex. Neither would her long-term relationship. As it was, Sophie had salvaged both relationships. Now, she claimed, she had the best of both worlds. She was no longer monogamous, she commented. But then she wasn't exactly non-monogamous, either. She paused a moment. "I've got it! I'm metamonogamous," she announced jubilantly.

The more we can resist the tidy resolution demanded by the togetherness story, the more we can enjoy new tales of mystery and intrigue. Meanwhile, lingering in the unknown zone gives us plenty of opportunity to play the sleuth in the continuing mystery of love and life. We discover, for example, that urgency is a brilliant bluffer and that, in fact, nothing terrible happens when we don't obey its imperial summons. We learn that erotic energy can be savored even when it isn't converted into caresses and kisses and that, left in its original form, it never burns out. And, ultimately, if we are patient enough, we learn to recognize new varieties of intimacy. Subtle, unique, each can occupy a special place in our lives. No choice has been necessary after all.

Practicing the art of the sequel may consist of lingering in the twilight zone between passion and permanence. But such intentional dawdling in uncharted regions may not suit everyone. For the less mystery minded among us, there are other ways to tell cliffhanger stories.

Another way of spinning out sequels is simply to go back and pick up the thread of an old story—one that has been a personal favorite of many of us ever since we first crawled, toddled, or pedaled off in search of that first big adventure.

Partnership and Peril: Finding the Right Balance

Accounts of lesbian girlhood are packed with the exploits of mini-Martinas and pint-sized Amelias, girls that outrun, outjump, outclimb, outsmart, and in short outadventure the boys. Even as grown-ups, plenty of lesbians are still sneaking past the sentinels posted in front of the boys-only adventure club. Our folk heroes regularly break world records and spearhead political movements, pen deathless prose and build cultural bridges.

For many of us, coming out has also been a kind of hero's journey. We barely squeak between Scylla and Charybdis, the crashing twin rocks of desire and dread. We creep past the Cyclops of parental scrutiny. We lose our rudders and compasses to the Sirens along the way, and, for what seems like eternity, we wander adrift. But at the same time, as we are sailing into the eye of the hurricane, we may also be falling in love.

As soon as the journey is over and we have reached our destination, it seems that the two aspects of our lives—love and adventure—fit snugly together. And they do for a while. After all, we have settled down with our one-and-only. Weeks, months, even years pass serenely. Too serenely. Until one day, we begin to feel restless. We begin to suspect that our desire to curl up together in front of the blazing fire and our yearning for on-the-edge vertigo are separate, not-terribly-compatible strands of our lives. The itch for a solo adventure may surface as a new attraction. Or, even more

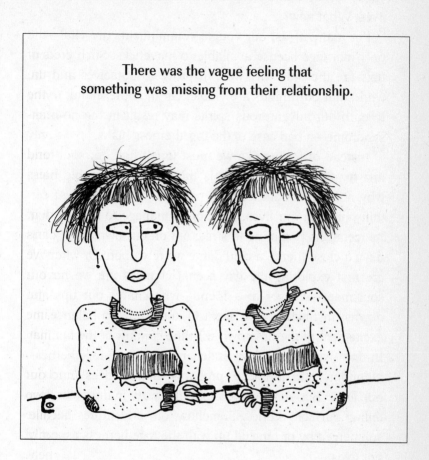

There was the vague feeling that
something was missing from their relationship.

commonly, the suppressed urge may come in the form of a vague feeling that something important is missing from our lives. What now?

For many of us, our couple commitments are vital—the only marriage license available to mavericks. Such credentials are the only way we can prove to ourselves and the world that our unions are viable. On the other hand, trying to curb our adventurous spirits may result in the ho-hum-syndrome—a bad case of the togetherness blahs.

Instead of feeling like we must forfeit half our soul (and just try figuring out which is the more dispensable half), why not make room for both partnership *and* peril? At certain points in our lives, most of us manage to do just that. As teenagers preparing to strike out on our own, most of us have a close friend, a confidante we rely upon. Or when we are first exploring the gay scene, chances are we have a soul mate—a lover or a friend—who shares our ups and downs. Instinctively we seem to know how to balance the excitement of the unknown with the comfort of the familiar. In fact, some blend of independence and togetherness, autonomy and intimacy, probably characterizes much of our lives. But somewhere along the way, many of us stop telling our solo stories. Somehow, our adventures become submerged by or tangled up with the togetherness aspect of our lives.

Take Sophie, for example. At first, her commitment to her partner and her desire for excitement seemed to be jumbled up in a hopeless mess. One way around the showdown between passion and partnership is to tell a new tale about the in-between sort of intimacy mentioned above. But there is another way out of this either/or dilemma. What if, for example, we see Sophie's responsiveness to Marta as a sign that the adventurous part of her life—dormant for years—is simply stirring again?

Within such a framework, trying to make a choice between her partner and her new flame becomes rather silly ... like trying to choose between seeing and hearing. Obviously, both are important. Instead of trying to choose between love and adventure, Sophie must find a way to separate the two very distinct strands of her life. And after she untangles them, she must find a way to give each its due.

If fact, Sophie's ongoing love story shows no signs of winding down. It is a story told collaboratively with her girlfriend during nightly pillow talk, daily phone calls from work, during anniversaries and birthdays and holidays. Even when they bicker over the acceptable levels of household hygiene, Sophie and her partner are invoking their shared history and foretelling a shared future together.

On the other hand, limerence is Sophie's adventure of choice. She's not unusual. For plenty of us, all adventures pale by comparison with the excitement of a new passion. But being swept away isn't the only mode of transport into the unknown.

There is no single recipe for risk taking. Some us of may limit ourselves to the pursuit of ecstasy. Others may prefer to grapple with private demons. Still others may want to tackle social ills. And for plenty of us, simply living through the day—or night—is adventure enough.

Lesbian True-Life Adventure Stories

There is no one-and-only adventure story. What would be suitably harrowing to some would be tedious to others. Still, despite their diversity, adventure stories share a common theme. In some unpredictable way, we are transformed by a curious combination of pleasure and danger. We know—sort of—who we are when we first embark on the adventure. But, at some point along the way, our most dearly held convictions begin to dissolve. Just how such personal quests can rearrange our molecules is clear from the following true adventure stories.

Claudia: Following Gulliver

Claudia had always been perfectly content when she lived alone. It was only after she moved in with Sid that she started feeling lonely. It was as though, quite abruptly, she had no one to talk to, no one who would dish a new film with her or compare notes on a novel. Sid, permanently parked in front of the TV, seemed oblivious to everything going on in the world around her. It was hard to say which was more frustrating—the fact that her twelfth graders or her lover refused to crack a book. But, there *was* one thing Claudia was sure of: something had to give.

The "something" came in the form of an application. The American Association of University Women was offering to pick up the tab for a special seminar. If you were one of the teachers who the selection committee deemed had a very good reason for wanting to become more proficient in English literature, you would win an all-expense-paid summer tutorial at Cambridge.

Claudia had a very good reason. Under the objectives section of the application, she spelled it out: "As an African American teacher in a school with a student body that is 99 percent non-Caucasian, I am always torn between teaching what is culturally relevant and most likely to boost my students' self-esteem, on the one hand and, on the other, what is Eurocentric and likely to help them get into college. I hope that participating in this seminar will help me find a way to bridge the gap between my students' lives and the work of the writers who, in their polite moments, my students refer to as 'dead white men.'"

When Claudia got word that out of hundreds of applicants she had been one of the handful chosen, she was elated . . . and then panic-stricken. She was frustrated with the status quo all right. But when it came right down to it, she was terrified of leaving Sidney for so long. She put her misgivings aside long enough to write a gracious acceptance letter.

The panicky feeling came back in the airport. Her hands got sweaty, and a voice began to throb in her head: "What are you doing going so far from home?" the critic who had taken up residence in her skull demanded to know. "Are you crazy?"

When Claudia saw her room at Cambridge, the panic intensified. Surely she couldn't be expected to sleep in the narrow, medieval pallet. And someone had neglected to remind the sun that it was July. She glanced around the walls of the barracks-like room. Not a thermostat in sight. Not even an electric blanket. But at least the window over her desk faced the courtyard. When, looking out, she found herself eyeball-to-eyeball with a leering gargoyle, she yanked down her shade, sat on her bed, and wept.

The common areas weren't much better. Meals were funereally sedate. After a grace, unidentifiable food was passed down the rows. She would have given her right arm for a chicken enchilada or, for that matter, anything that looked and tasted faintly familiar.

But the seminar, itself. Ahh, now that was something else. If the professor never exactly resurrected the dead white men, she certainly breathed life into the culture that produced them. Nothing was off-limits. They discussed the hair styles and sewage problems and sexual peccadilloes of Shakespeare and his contemporaries. They eavesdropped on the gossip of long-ago London, hobnobbed with the homeless and the highborn. And on the last day of the seminar, all the students were invited to a potluck in the professor's home. The only requirement: each of them had to come in sixteenth-century costume and bring a dish of the day. With a blanket and a bit of rope, Claudia managed to improvise a cassock. A jug of sour beer and a hunk of rye bread provided the perfect finishing touches to her friar ensemble.

She missed Sidney terribly. And yet, at the same time, Sid seemed to be part of another world, a different lifetime. And Claudia began to see how she could make connections that her students would get: links between Gulliver and Captain Kirk, or Othello and O.J.

But, of course, this was what she had come for, what she had expected would happen. What she hadn't expected was her homecoming. Stacked on Sidney's desk were books. Dozens of them. Everything by Morrison and Baldwin. Even the latest novel by Sapphire. While Claudia had been away, Sidney had been conducting her own seminar. And now she wanted to talk.

Lover ennui is not a sign that something is wrong at home. It simply means we have neglected another, equally vital, part of our life stories. And if we are resourceful and determined enough, our adventure stories don't have to be told at the expense of forever-after. Free-form or prepackaged, our exploits may last a day or a lifetime. They may require chutzpah or stamina, a willingness to journey down deep inside ourselves or to apply a new design on the surface of our lives.

Cicely: Adventure in the Skin Trade

Cicely had a partner she was crazy about, three slavishly devoted dogs, one mean-spirited Siamese, a turtle, and a parakeet. There they all were, in the process of living happily ever after, when Cicely got restless. She needed something more . . . but what? An affair? She dismissed it as too complicated. A baby perhaps? Too time-consuming. Finally, the answer came to her when she was gridlocked in her usual morning commute: what she really wanted was a tattoo. Not some wimpy butterfly or star tucked away underneath a bra strap or peeping out of a panty line, so concealed that only her partner would know. No, she wanted something gaudy and gorgeous. Something that no nurse would be caught dead sporting. Something that would blow her patients' minds.

Unfortunately, it was her lover whose mind was blown. Ronni was a probation officer. Tattoos freaked her out. All she could picture were dripping hearts, circled with barbed wire, or scantily clad babes, their breasts bulging whenever her parolees flexed their biceps.

When all her attempts to broaden Ronni's horizons degenerated into fights, Cicely realized that she was never going to get Ronni's blessing. If she wanted a tattoo, she had to go ahead on her own.

She approached her adventure as methodically as a graduate student preparing for orals: she researched her subject. Thoroughly. She read about the history of tattoos and their cultural significance in different times and places. She pored over the memoirs of tattoo artists and subscribed to magazines for tattoo connoisseurs. She even started going to tattoo conventions.

Next came the decal stage. Before she did something irreversible, she wanted to see how such a public display felt. Ronni was an amateur botanist. Cicely figured her lover would be less likely to recoil in horror if her first faux attempts were floral.

For the next six months, Cicely applied roses, violets, orchids to her arms and legs. When they wore off, she replaced them with new bouquets and garlands.

Though the decals only elicited more horrified eye rolling from Ronni, Cicely decided she liked the feeling of being an ambulatory artwork. And by this time, she had seen enough tattoos to settle on an artist and a design. She wanted a cobra. And she wanted Julie Moon, one of the few internationally respected women artists, to tattoo the serpent on her arm on the morning of her thirty-fifth birthday.

The prickling sensations continued for hours. But when Julie finally put down her needles and Cicely opened her eyes, she was thrilled. Undulating from her wrist to her elbow was a vibrant green and lavender reptile. With its flared hood, extended tongue, and spiking tail, it was both menacing and seductive.

And her lover? Ronni never exactly came around. But then, she could hardly disapprove of such magnificent beastliness. Now Cicely is trying to decide what to put on her other arm. And after that, who knows?

Adventures come in all shapes and sizes. And sometimes it is impossible to figure out which is the *real* cliffhanger: pursuing a private dream or waiting to see if your partner will stick around while you try to make it come true.

Carmen: A Will-She-or-Won't-She Cliffhanger

As a child Carmen had loved holding her younger brothers and sisters, dressing them, roughhousing with them. And although she had always wanted her own kid, she had kissed that possibility good-bye when she kissed her first woman lover. But years had passed. Times had changed. Now that several of her lesbian friends were in the process

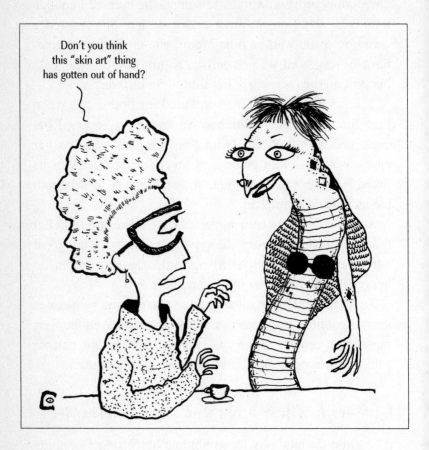

of becoming parents, she, too, could envision the possibility. More than envision it. She ached for it. But there was one obstacle.

After half a dozen false starts, she had finally found the right woman. Hokey as it sounded, she hoped she would grow old with Betsy. Even though they lived an hour apart, they spent every free minute together. They loved each other's company. They liked each other's friends and families and the same kind of leisurely, sun-drenched vacations. They even both liked the same brand of vanilla sex. They were a perfect match—soul mates in every respect except one.

The last thing in the world Betsy wanted was a kid. Her objections were all perfectly reasonable. They were already both too busy. And raising a child was expensive. There would be no money left over for fun. And what about sex? Surely the patter of little feet outside the bedroom door was not anyone's idea of an aphrodisiac. Besides, there were already too many people in the world.

At least Carmen had an answer to this last objection. She would adopt.

It didn't matter. Betsy remained adamant. No kids. Period. Ever. Afraid of what the answer might be, Carmen never asked whether Betsy would break up with her if and when the baby arrived. She only said quietly that the parenting responsibilities for the child would be hers alone. And that she hoped that, in time, Betsy would come to have some kind of relationship with the new addition.

Then Carmen started her campaign. Every adoption agency in the country received a packet that contained her autobiography, photos of her playing with her nieces and nephews, and testimonials about her maternal potential from everyone who knew her. The packet even included a floor plan of the house with an X marking the room that would be converted to the newcomer's bedroom.

It took a year to get a nibble. It came from a single mom who already had a five- and seven-year-old. Her third child, two-year-old Esperanza, was stretching her to the limit. Esperanza's mother, Teresa, liked the idea that another single mom, like herself, would be raising Espy.

Over the next six months, Carmen visited Teresa and her family several times. And then she brought Espy back to her home in Los Angeles. What was supposed to be a short visit stretched into a month, and then two. When Carmen finally took Espy back to San Jose, it was only to sign the papers and say good-bye.

All of Betsy's predictions came true. Everything changed. Money and sex got much scarcer. Their Hawaiian vacations had to be scaled back to overnight campouts in the back-yard. But Carmen was radiant, and Espy . . . well, Espy was a great kid. In time, even Betsy had to admit the trade-off was worth it.

Sometime in our lives, most of us dream about accomplishing something special. We promise ourselves we will make the world a better place to live in or take a sabbatical from work and bum around the world for a year or sequester ourselves long enough to become the artists or writers we have always claimed to be. Unfortunately, it usually takes a breakup for us to reclaim the half-a-soul we have forfeited. Think of how valuable such adventures might be if we were to undertake them when we were still partnered. True, they may be nerve-racking; yet, in the end, such adventures can strengthen our relationships.

Togetherness is a sweet, even necessary, tale. We know it so well, we can recite it in our sleep. But when it is the only story we get to hear or tell, it turns into a straitjacket, confining our imaginations *and* our intimacies.

When it comes to our lives and loves, we need a generous supply of alternative stories: instructive sci-fi fables and twilight-zone mysteries, endless sequels and white-knuckle exploits. We are both hearth huggers *and* voyagers. We must make room in our lives for the dream of forever-after and the determination to never look back.

Sophie: A Postscript

It *is* possible to be committed to a partner and still have intense feelings about someone new. But preventing such adventures from getting tangled up with an ongoing togetherness tale or, worse yet, turning into a new one, requires skill and nerve.

If we elect to experiment with such perilous pleasures, we need to become comfortable with disorientation. We'll have to tolerate long stretches of it. And perhaps most important, we have to be able to tell our own to-be-continued love stories when our partners are embarking on their own solo adventures.

Chapter 6

Jealousy for Beginners: Taming the Green-Eyed Monster

When it comes to The Other Woman stories, most of us have a mother-of-all-mayhem favorite: the trusted friend who turned out to be a snake; the cute new shortstop who made her best plays without benefit of ball or glove; the sultry Ms. Subaru who tried to borrow your girlfriend along with the lug wrench.

Tales of such dangerous intruders pepper our collective history as well. Thanks to her rivals, Sappho had plenty of opportunity to sharpen her ice-pick wit. And where would dyke drama be without the legendary bed hopping of Natalie Barney and Renee Vivian, Vita Sackville-West and Violet Trefusis? Even the indefatigable conjugality of Gertrude and Alice is rumored to have been ruffled regularly by visits from Mabel Dodge Luhan, a free-spirited flirt with literary leanings.

Jealousy can, and often does, convert perfectly routine domesticity into a lurid blockbuster, a juggernaut that instantly muscles every other story about love and life out of its path. Should we ever require proof of the absolute tyranny of such tales, we need only check our own racing pulse, dilated pupils, and sweaty palms during a meltdown. Once in the embrace of the green-eyed monster, there is no going back. In fact, often it is the she-done-me-wrong storyteller—not her perfidious mate—who initiates divorce proceedings. A straying partner may have no intention of eloping with a temporary divertissement. According to the version favored by her prematurely grieving partner, however, the infidel has already disappeared into the sunset, new inamorata in tow.

Why is sexual jealousy so convincing—so able to wipe out, in a flash, years of devotion? There is no dearth of explanations for jealousy's visceral wallop. Exponents of the survival-of-the-fittest school believe, for example, that our panicky reaction to possible loss is biologically hardwired, the evolutionary legacy of billions of years: the more jittery our mammalian ancestors, the louder the squeals. The bigger the commotion, the more likely foraging mothers or mates would come to the rescue before the predators arrived. Those who didn't squeak up quickly became cougar plat du jour; their panicky but surviving brothers and sisters, the passed-on gene de Pleistocene.

Plenty of us don't have to peek through the prehistoric foliage of Jurassic Park for a glimpse of the green-eyed monster. We have only to conjure up our own childhoods for an explanation of jealousy's souped-up potency. Having always been the apple of our parents' eyes, perhaps we resented being pared down to the core by the new arrival. To add insult to injury, we were then pressed into service as baby-sitter, cook, and bottle washer. Thereafter, our undiminished howls of protest have never been far from the surface.

Or perhaps our induction into the jealousy club didn't occur until later in life. Being new lesbians on the block, we never questioned the relationship sequence summarized succinctly on a recent Internet bulletin board:

1. Thing/item/date
2. Boink
3. Commitment

Nobody mentioned that after a year or two or three, there would be someone else. Or that new boink would mean goink goink gone. Now, the mere hint of another intruder sends us into a frenzy. It matters little which theory we subscribe to. They all boil down to one conclusion: most of us believe that our overheated reaction to potential rivals is inevitable, something we can't change. Fueled by earthshaking events beyond our control, jealousy is bound to whipsaw us back and forth like palms in the path of a hurricane.

Angst Anonymous, Anyone?

Perhaps it is true that our jealousy-sensitized nerve endings have been programmed by some combination of nature and (absence of) nurture. Yet, couldn't we make the same claim about any strong emotion? Take anger, for example. Fury can be just as primal, as overdetermined by genetic design or family feuds. Ah, but here is where the difference between jealousy and other emotional tsunamis becomes painfully obvious.

In contrast to the wildly jealous, the passionately pissed off have choices about how to react—a whole menu of parables to choose from. There are, of course, out-of-control outbursts, thunderclaps that can rival any jealousy firestorm we can imagine. Still, there are plenty of other options: being assertive or aggressive; getting it off your chest or stuffing it; stewing or denial; subtle sulking or even displacing your wrath on the hapless driver in front of you. And for the serious ragers, the batterers who seem to know only one story, the social pressure is intense: diversify those limited parable portfolios, or else! Many urban areas provide resources that do just that: support groups, individual therapy, self-help techniques. After learning to count to ten, breathe deeply, take time-outs, and visualize soothing scenes, several bash-prone individuals I've known have even been reborn as Zen masters—enlightened as well as transformed.

Just think what might happen if those of us gripped by the green-eyed monster had access to such a repertoire of jealousy management strategies? What if we could find relief in Angst Anonymous, call hot lines set up for terror of abandonment, consult with psychics who specialize in "other woman" exorcisms? What if we could even buy panic zippers to go along with our worry beads?

If we had an entire infrastructure similar to the one many of us use to deal with domestic violence, sexual abuse, and alcohol or drug problems, we could learn a whole new jealousy repertoire and soon be able to tell tales of reorientation and restraint, of transformation and cure.

Instead, there is . . . nothing. A resounding silence. Or worse, the reinforcement of the meltdown saga. With forever-after thrumming so relentlessly in our hearts and minds, the first hint of partner slippage becomes a matter of life and death, honor, pride, survival. No wonder our sexual jealousy stories always turn into do-or-die epics.

That means it's up to us. Since there are no helping hands, no structured community support for jealousy recovery, we must design our own program. The first step is simple. We have to start collecting alternatives to the meltdown epic.

Rehab programs designed for rage-aholics start with just such downsized stories. Those who feel like victims of out-of-control anger learn to notice the nuances, the different degrees and states of vexation. For example, feeling peevish qualifies as anger, but, on the scale, it is far from "going ballistic." A small irritation is light-years away from all-out wrath.

The same sort of variations exist within jealousy. Sometimes we may find ourselves in a prejealous state of

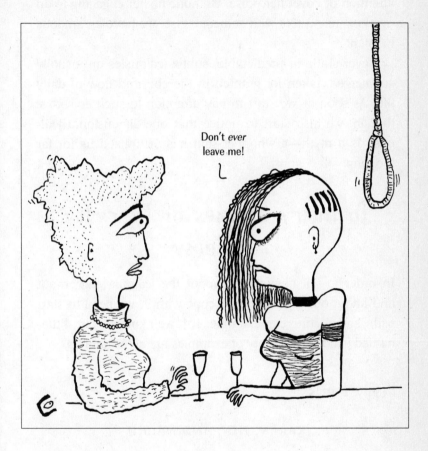

uneasiness or self-doubt. Sometimes, during a social event, we may feel left out. Perhaps we yearn for our partner's attention or covet her poise. Or, noticing her engaging in an overlong tête-à-tête with someone else, we have an anxious moment.

Never static or predictable, subtle jealousies are usually submerged, taken for granted in the ebb and flow of daily life. As soon as we start to pay attention to such episodes, though, we also start to notice that one-dimensional jealousy is a myth—a whopper that has victimized us for far too long.

Ordinary Stories of Everyday Jealousy

In order to tell new stories about the jealousy juggernaut and about our own ability to cope with it, we need to start with some concrete examples of well-known but little-named jealousies. Plenty of examples are all around us.

Puppy Pangs

KAREN, JIIN, AND NACHO

Karen never slept through the night. If her asthma didn't wake her up, her old shoulder injury would. She would toss and turn until, surrendering to the inevitable, she would hunt for the Advil PM. Because such nocturnal episodes tended to disturb her partner, Jiin, both had decided that they should sleep apart for a while. They were still spending nights in separate rooms when Karen decided to adopt Nacho, the only female from a neighborhood litter of apricot-colored pups. After Nacho arrived, Karen didn't sleep alone anymore. Jiin, who had been the one to suggest the separate arrangement in the first place, began to feel lonely and left out. She was horrified to think she was jealous of a dog and even more horrified one morning, when she found Karen and Nacho in bed together snuggling, to hear herself blurt out, "You love that dog more than me!"

The most common other woman in lesbian relationships is most likely not a lesbian, not even a Homo sapiens. Feathered or furred, the new arrival usually doesn't hide its profound preference for one member of the couple. Or its dislike of the other member. A client who often looked as though she had been mugged told me that her partner's parrot was the culprit. It never failed to lunge at her, claws extended, beak at the ready, whenever they were in the same room.

A friend of mine tells me that Bingo, her Manx, rolls around quite deliberately in a nearby barnyard. After his fur is suitably freighted with chicken droppings and miscellaneous ca-ca, he makes a beeline for the side of the bed occupied every night by my friend's lover. There he molts and marinates until forcibly removed.

To make matters worse, when wounded and affronted partners complain about the interspecies love affairs occurring under their noses, typically they are ridiculed by the

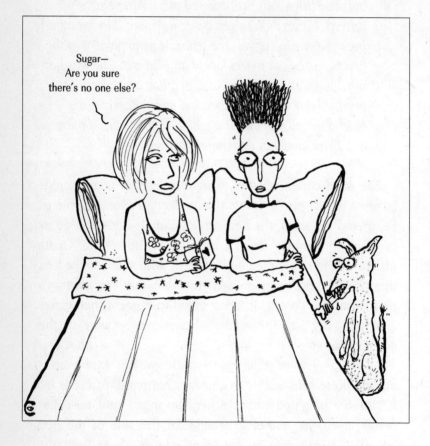

human member of the liaison. In spite of the derision and denial, partners of pet lovers know perfectly well who, in case of a burning house or other emergency, will be rescued first.

Ex-Lover Pique

Interestingly enough, it is not only pets who compete with partners for the alpha lover's slot. Ex-lovers can also be serious contenders.

AJA, TREVOR, AND CINDY

Aja and Trevor started an affair before Trev had broken up with Cindy, her previous lover. At the time, Trev reassured Aja that the old relationship, nonsexual and comfortable as an old shoe, had been a marriage of convenience for years. It was just that neither had had the guts to give it the final coup de grace. Now five years into their relationship, Aja isn't sure if the old relationship ever really ended after all. Trev calls Cindy every day, includes her in every holiday and vacation, and taps the pool of household funds whenever Cindy needs financial help. If Aja protests, Trev just shrugs and invokes Cindy's unassailably sacred status as "family."

After interviewing dozens of lesbian ex-lovers, psychologist Carol Becker wrote a book about postpartnership connection. The title of the book—*Unbroken Ties*—sums up her findings.

The strength of ex-lovers' attachments may not be evident right after a separation. Following breakups, many of us remain too raw to agree to anything more than shared dog custody. But after enough time passes, old betrayals and disappointments lose some of their sting. When enough memories of the good old days resurface, one ex or the other is likely to make a friendly overture. According to one national survey, more than 60 percent of lesbians become friends with their exlovers. Author Becker suggests that the postbreakup relationships often evolve into what many of us refer to as family.

At first glance, these chosen families seem like great improvements over the blood relatives who generally have been only too happy to saw the queer branch off the family tree. Indeed, our well-tested postbreakup relationships are often a blessing. But, positive as they seem, they can also raise thorny issues for ongoing twosomes.

Both positive and problematic sides of ex-lover relationships are evident in the lifelong attachment of anthropologists Margaret Mead and Ruth Benedict. Even after their love affair had lost momentum and both were established in new relationships, they kept in close touch with each other. Over the next twenty years, they corresponded regularly and rendezvoused periodically. They midwifed each other's careers and supported each other in times of trouble. After Benedict's death, Mead was generally acknowledged to be the chief mourner and central relationship of Benedict's life. One can only surmise what Ruth Valentine, Benedict's domestic partner at the time, felt about her exclusion from the small circle of the openly bereft.

The more one member of a couple cherishes her previous partner, the more likely the ex will be perceived as a rival by the other half of the couple. The current partner may feel that she and her lover's ex are both contending for the same finite supply of intimacy and affection.

Of course, reactions to ex-lover bonds vary enormously. Some women are only too glad that their partner has someone else to lean on, while others keep the "ex-lovers unwelcome" mat permanently on display. The most common reaction of one partner to her lover's past partner probably hovers somewhere between approval and animosity. We might label this midway point "ex-lover pique." Partners afflicted by such pique claim it is short-lived, a transient state provoked when they happen to overhear casual endearments slip out during a phone conversation between the two onetime lovers or witness a display of easy affection during a greeting.

Ex-lover pique can be triggered by other factors. Often onetime lovers have bonds that go beyond their shared history. Perhaps both old lovers came of age in the political turbulence of the sixties. Perhaps both happen to be the oldest daughters in Irish Catholic families. By accident of birth, the more current partner becomes an automatic outsider, permanently exiled from membership in the special club the ex-lovers share.

Ex-lover pique can be annoying. But unlike other forms of jealousy, it can serve a very positive purpose—an intermittent and necessary reminder that, much as we might want to, we can't be all things to a lover.

Posttraumatic Jealousy

We might call ex-lover pique "functional" jealousy. In contrast, another type of jealousy—the posttraumatic variety—has nothing redeeming about it. Posttraumatic jealousy is also sparked by ex-lovers. But in this case the visitors from the past appear strictly in flashback form.

MARYBETH AND JACKIE

Marybeth's new lover was nothing like her ex. For starters, Jackie was perfectly content. It was obvious that she had no desire to run away with anyone else. But even though Marybeth kept reminding herself of Jackie's commitment, it didn't matter. If Jackie was unexpectedly late or sounded distracted during a phone call, Marybeth would start to lose it. Once the panic button had been pressed, she was sure Jackie was staying late so she could have coffee with a co-worker. While they were becoming more than just colleagues, Marybeth imagined them flirting or plotting a more serious rendezvous.

Marybeth tried to reason with herself. All to no avail. It was only after Jackie came home exhausted, raving about an extralong meeting, that Marybeth was able to shake herself out of her trance.

After a previous lover has decamped with someone new, the abandoned partner often suffers acute bouts of both loss and jealousy. Eventually the two feelings become permanently fused—interlocking emotional events. For years to come, neither feeling can occur independently of the other. After a traumatic breakup, jealousy must forever be a preview of loss, just as loss is the inevitable aftermath of jealousy. The combination is particularly deadly.

After a painful breakup, the brokenhearted know the anatomy of betrayal by heart. They have memorized the delays, excuses, and denials favored by an about-to-defect lover. Unfortunately, it is very hard to distinguish between the evasive maneuvers of a straying mate and ordinary mishaps. Even perfectly innocent partners get caught in traffic jams, have headaches, and sound distracted from time to time.

Once in new relationships, the walking wounded realize that they have lost the ability to distinguish between ominous cues and ordinary contretemps. They scramble to compensate. These reparation attempts give posttraumatic jealousy its special flavor. At the same time as the love-shocked are convinced abandonment is imminent, they are delivering keep-cool lectures to themselves: don't be silly; that was then, this is now. But part of them remains unconvinced. Icy logic combined with adrenalized dread characterizes posttraumatic jealousy.

Bleed-Through Jealousy

Those who suffer from posttraumatic jitters rarely feel in control. In contrast, another form of jealousy is most commonly experienced by those who never feel out of control. Bleed-through jealousy tends to penetrate the most carefully constructed defenses.

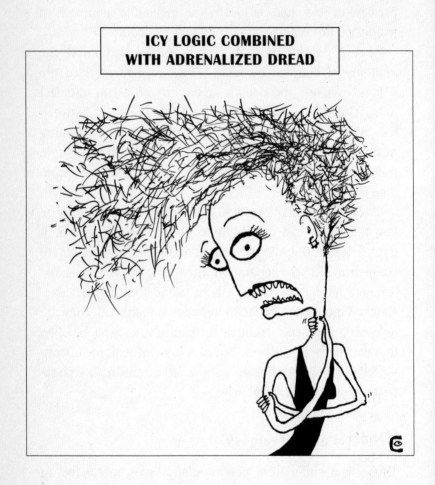

ICY LOGIC COMBINED
WITH ADRENALIZED DREAD

RANI AND NAT

Rani and Nat told themselves they were rare: one of the special couples who had managed to avoid all the usual possessive traps. Not only were they jealousy free, they actually enjoyed hearing about each other's adventures with other women. Perhaps, they speculated, it was simply that neither had ever met anyone who actually threatened their relationship.

As it turned out, the half-expected threat never materialized. Instead, a rather banal coincidence ended their complacency.

On one of their prearranged days off, Rani decided to go shopping. Starting down the produce aisle, she stopped short. There were Nat and her other lover, standing close to each other whispering, laughing, jiggling, and sniffing cantaloupes in an attempt to find a ripe one. For Rani, it was a glimpse of unbearable intimacy, a sort of flagrante delicto much more painful than anything she might have witnessed had she caught them in bed.

Those of us who have opted for multiple relationships have labored hard and long to overcome conventional conditioning. Why, the antimonogamy argument goes, should full-bodied, physical expression of interest or caring be limited to one person? Or as the slogan on one popular T-shirt reads: So many women, so little time.

With the same unflagging reasonableness, the nonmonogamists set up rules to control traffic between their loves. They hope that the establishment of clear boundaries—

who, when, where, and what—will protect everyone concerned from undue jealousy. But in an unguarded moment— a glimpse of a partner straightening her other lover's collar or sharing a private joke—it becomes apparent that something has escaped the rules. Unnamed, it can't be contained and controlled. Despite all understandings, two lovers have managed to escape to the timeless place that only intimates share. For the excluded partner, the pain of the realization is both sudden and sharp.

Those of us who claim to be jealousy free are talented storytellers. And if one story fails us, we usually set to work crafting a new one. Perhaps we find a way to discount the intimacy we accidentally witnessed, or we craft a superintimacy, an exalted closeness that our partners share with no one but ourselves. Yet, after we have had one episode of bleed-through jealousy, it's much easier to have a second and a third. Our old walk-on-water equanimity is never quite the same again.

Poison Ivy Jealousy

The nonmonogamous have their own unique varieties of jealously. Poison ivy jealousy is more chronic than the bleed-through type—more like a perpetual itch than an unexpected blast.

TESS AND AUDRE

It didn't seem quite fair. Audre never had a shortage of dates. Introverted, shy, Tess had never been able to

*generate the same volume of outside possibilities. So
there she was on Saturday night, watching her once-
and-future girlfriend put together the perfect outfit—the
vest that matched the green flecks in her eyes, the blouse
that revealed just the right amount of cleavage. And
when she was finally alone with the cats and the TV,
there was no rush of panic, no slash-and-burn fantasy.
Instead, Tess was just restless. It was impossible for her
to get comfortable anywhere.*

If anyone should have been able to defang the green-
eyed monster, it is the lesbians who have declared multiple
lovers a lifestyle. Such erotic adventurers are not unique to
our times or even to Lesbian Nation. Proponents of free
love in the twenties, swingers in the sixties, and polyamorists in the nineties, they defy easy classification. They can
be gay, straight, or bi; married, single, or communally clustered. Their only common denominator is their nonmonogamous credo.

A polyamorist magazine, *Loving More,* is full of tips about
where to meet like-minded people, anecdotes about casual
affairs, and suggestions for how to build more enduring
polyamorous families. And, surprise, how to deal with jealousy!

Far from avoiding the usual abandonment jitters,
polyamorists get just as nervous as most monogamists. But
here's another eye opener. Rather than trying to purge
either the other woman or the unsettling emotion,
polyamorists seem to have pegged jealousy as a manageable form of madness—a devilish case of emotional poison

ivy that every now and then gets the better of them. Some of the victims of the pernicious itch just squirm or white-knuckle their way through the ordeal. The less stoic sub-scribers to the jealousy-as-controllable-rash perspective tend to ask for calamine lotion in the form of extra reassur-ance, or they go back to the drawing board to craft new remedies or rules.

On the surface, dykes who want multiple partners seem to differ from the monogamists in many ways. Perhaps they crave more novelty or meet their security needs in more roundabout ways. But the major difference between the two groups has to do with jealousy. Unlike the monogamists, the poly crowd believes that jealousy, rather like death and taxes, is a normal rather than abnormal state—a feeling to be managed instead of a rival to be murdered.

Mother Envy

Another multiple relationship—the one that exists between two lesbian parents and their child—is likely to generate another sort of maddening, if manageable, emotional rash.

NYAMI, TARA, AND ANGELA

They had been forewarned. Long before making the first appointment at the sperm bank, they were reconciled to the prospect of having a boy. So, when Angela arrived, she seemed like a gift from the goddess, an olive-eyed, velvety-limbed miracle. Despite sleep deprivation, diaper rash, colic, and child care dilemmas, the couple's delight continued undiminished. That is, until Angie started babbling.

"Ma Ma Ma," Angela would gurgle, looking inquiringly from Nyami to Tara.

Who was Mama going to be? They had never spelled it out, but Tara assumed their previous fifty-fifty partnership would continue.

Nyami saw it differently. "No way. She's going to be confused enough about who she is with no dad, with one black and one white woman raising her. She is not going to be confused about who her mother is."

"Where's the law that says she can't have two mothers?" retorted Tara. "I'm her mother, too."

After a week of wrangling they reached a compromise: they would be, respectively, Mama and Mama-Tara. For the most part it worked. But it always hurt Tara when Angela, after a bad dream or a scuffed knee, could be comforted only by Mama.

Lesbian co-motherhood requires teamwork. Mothers-to-be have to support each other through rejections from friends and family and resistance from courts and the medical establishment. Yet even after so much us-against-them practice, lesbian moms often end up on opposing teams. How does it happen?

The basis for the eventual rift starts in girlhood. No sooner are most of us out of diapers than our mother-in-training apprenticeship begins. Without any separate and clear-cut roles to prevent overlap—even competition—between ace nurturers, two child-rearing specialists must use ingenuity to carve out separate nest-tending functions. Sometimes mothering duties sort easily into, say, night and day shifts. Or perhaps one mom takes charge of feeding and clothes, while the other mom manages bath and bowels.

But the cultural script about motherhood is very insistent. No matter how well intentioned and inventive they are, partners may begin to struggle, secretly or openly, about who gets to be the "real" mom. For the non-biological-mother, the odds aren't good. Both law and custom reinforce the legitimacy of the birth mother's role. Adding to the precariousness of the non-birth mother's position is the likelihood that the biological mother is smitten with the newborn. Perhaps she is already entertaining fantasies of eloping with "her" baby. The non-bio-mom may worry that, if she pushes too hard for her fair share of motherhood, she may find herself minus a kid *and* a partner.

Inequality and mother envy go hand in hand. Of course, power imbalances are not only due to discrepancies in parenting roles. One partner may have an entirely different sort of leverage—she may control the time the partners spend together.

Time Possessiveness

Potential rivals are the sort of hot spots we expect in any relationship. More startling, yet increasingly common, is a type of jealousy provoked by an entirely different source. In a world of ever-tightening schedules, the struggle for possession of a partner's time can be even more challenging than any attempt to keep her heart.

DECCA AND LOURDES

Decca's pot-growing days were far behind her. During those long-ago cash-rich years, however, she had bought enough rental real estate to be self-sufficient. Now her time was hers to manage as she wished. Figuring it was community payback time, she spent her days volunteering as a drug rehab counselor. Evenings were reserved for dog walks and friends, for films, and for Lourdes, her girlfriend.

In contrast, every minute of Lourdes's time was spoken for, several times over. She got up at dawn every day to commute to her Silicon Valley job. Nights and weekends were devoted to getting the law degree that she hoped would liberate her from the corporate grind. AA meetings, friends, a bevy of sisters had to be squeezed into the little remaining time. And, of course, Decca.

On one of the precious Sunday afternoons Lourdes arranged to visit her family, Decca would try not to sulk. But, at the last minute, she would stand mutely at the door, looking beseechingly at Lourdes. Lourdes called it her Oliver Twist "more, please" look.

We tick off the bottom-line requirements of our relationship—intimacy, communication, sex—without really noticing that there is a much more basic ingredient: time together. Without a protected temporal zone, touching or even talking is impossible. Yet for many women—working, going to school, raising kids—time together is a perpetually deferred event, wishful thinking about a distant future when they can get away for a weekend. Often, however, both partners are not equally booked. The less-scheduled partner may be able to cadge twenty minutes after work to gaze into space or talk to friends. After she has had her dose of me-time, she is ready to be intimate with her partner. In fact, in her mind, her partner's first free moments are already reserved for the two of them.

The first jealous jab comes if the latecomer gives her a perfunctory peck and proceeds to read the paper or check her mail. On the other hand, if the busier partner jumps into the relationship as soon as she comes home, she bypasses her own private homecoming rituals. Her lover may be more content, but the busier woman is likely to start feeling hungry for her own alone time.

Time jealousy is frustrating. But it is also an important signal. It reminds us that someone or something—ourselves, our bosses, or just life in general—is imposing an impossible volume of demands on our time. Unless we clone ourselves, there is no way to do it all. Time jealousy is something to pay attention to. We might view it as an ailing canary in the mine shaft of an overbooked life. But rather than staying mindful of the larger schedule problem, one partner frequently tries to solve it herself—often with disastrous results.

The partner who is more jealous of her partner's time—and has more of the precious commodity herself—may become the gofer, chef, and housecleaner. By absorbing these tasks, she hopes her partner will be able to spend the little available time she has with her. Such solutions usually backfire. Liberated from household tasks, the overbooked partner may spend her extra moments curled up with a book. But even in situations where one partner's assumption of extra chores does provide more together time, such a role shift creates a problem down the road. As soon as the less busy partner becomes the de facto guardian of home and hearth, the other partner becomes the partner-with-the-precious time by default. Now the stage is set for another sort of jealousy.

Artificially Fortified Jealousy

Attempts to cure jealousy often only succeed in strengthening it. And in certain cases, so-called jealousy remedies act very much like pesticides. They may be effective in the short run. In the long run, however, they create super-pests—green-eyed monsters too powerful to rout.

HELEN AND TISH

Helen and Tish often joked that someone should nominate them as poster exes. Even during their breakup, they never flagged in their devotion. And afterward they remained the best of friends. When one went out of town, the other minded her pets and plants. They brought each other chicken soup during flu bouts and commiserated when new relationships hit the skids. Then one day Helen met Cassie. After they became lovers, the ensuing sparks flew far enough to ignite another fire. Tish, who had never been possessive before, felt her first jealous rush. When they all got together for dinner, Tish made no effort to hide her disdain for Cassie.

Cassie responded in kind. Thereafter, whenever either Tish or Cassie was alone with Helen, she spared no attempt to assassinate her rival's character.

Helen thought the solution was simple: more contact. Once they got to know each other better, she was certain, things would calm down. With such a détente in mind, she proposed they all go away for a weekend camping trip. Cassie and Tish agreed reluctantly.

The first night, after a cookout and a bottle of Chianti on the beach, Cassie and Helen went into their tent. Tish crawled in after them.

The three-way turned out to be a disaster. The familiarity of the two ex-lovers was more than Cassie could stomach. The new lovers' passion made Tish's heart sink. Helen was trying so hard to make everyone feel good that she ended up feeling like a geisha. On the way home, no one spoke. Instead of minimizing jealousy, the trip had given both Tish and Cassie just the pictures they needed to make it worse.

Direct assaults on jealousy rarely work. And the consequences of these attempts at cure usually exacerbate the problem. We come away from such "failures" with the story about jealousy's megapower artificially enhanced. We are now convinced that once the green-eyed monster gains momentum, we are at its mercy. After all, we tried. We did our best. And despite our efforts, the big J proved too much for us. The monster we have created by trying to fight jealousy is a much more formidable creature than ever before.

And, after our unsuccessful last stand, we are convinced that we are forever fated to be its helpless victims.

Jealousy remedies don't work for a simple reason. There is no such thing as jealousy.

Anatomy of a Whopper

The biggest whopper of them all concerns the green-eyed monster itself. Imposing, terrifying, something most of us want to avoid at all costs. But what if it is not even real? What if jealousy is a figment of someone's imagination—an invention like pi or the international dateline? If you think about it for a minute, it's pretty obvious that what we refer to as jealousy is just a point, and a pretty arbitrary point at that, on a continuum of feeling. After a certain amount of doubt, suspicion, and worry accumulates, we have an aha moment. "That's it!" we say to ourselves. "Of course. I must be jealous."

At first, this simple explanation for all that queasiness provides a welcome clarity, the equivalent of a lighthouse beacon slicing through the foggy turbulence. And if the very same set of feelings intensifies even more—and it often does—we are well on our way past jealousy and on to desperation.

But what if we start to notice that all the emotional states we label jealousy are different from one another? Some jealousies feature galloping self-doubts. Others are more characterized by rival-anxiety. Some are major obsessions, trumpeted from rooftops. Still others are quietly hoarded secrets.

And there are many shades of prejealousy as well. When a beloved's attention is diverted, we may feel uneasy or off-center. But we haven't yet reached the aha stage. Oh, shoot, we say to ourselves, if only she were lighting up like a Christmas tree over me instead of the pea-brained poodle or that space case of an ex-love.

Our reactions to these prejealousy states are as diverse as our personalities. Feeling a bit displaced, some of us call a friend to complain. If we are more assertive, we get in the faces of our distracted partners. The more athletically inclined just jog for an extra mile or two. Workaholics spend extra time doing what everyone assures them they do best. The more suggestible among us rent an underdog-triumphs-over-all video and identify fiercely with the improbable heroine. And, last but not least, the vindictive just plot small revenges. (Next time Fido's mistress goes out of town, he will—teehee—simply have to go on that long-overdue diet!)

In themselves, none of these rebalancing strategies is particularly significant. What is important is that we know how to soothe ourselves. Most of us change the distressing channel without fanfare. Without even realizing what we are doing, we activate mood-changing strategies developed long before we even got into our current relationship.

Most of us grow up with a plentiful supply of not-good-enough stories about ourselves. Vintage tales, they are left over from the miserable Saturday afternoon when we were the last kid chosen for a neighborhood kickball team or the time we flunked algebra or relationships 101. It's easy for a partner's preoccupation to reactivate old stories about our last-picked, least-wanted status. But after we've been around the block enough times, we learn where a different kickball team is forming. And this one will make us the captain. Perhaps the new "team" consists of a backup supply of good friends or a talent for getting lost in books. In any case, most of us have figured out some way to change the not-so-good stories about ourselves into tales that showcase our competence, style, and smarts.

Big J is a story, too. Unfortunately, it mimics the old not-good-enough story so closely that in a sense we are hypnotized. We forget that in the years since we got picked last, we have learned to how to undo old humiliations. We have figured out how to change the scene, to get strokes from another source. All our hard-won strategies forgotten, we slip back in the old neighborhood. Standing there shifting from one foot to the other, we get passed over again and again. We see the dismissive looks, feel the knot of despair growing in our stomachs. Hypnotized by the myth of J power, we don't rent *Revenge of the Nerds*, don't even bother to put on our magic jogging shoes that will carry us up, up, and away.

Even though there is no single remedy for jealousy, there is a way to undermine the hypnotic power of the J-myth. Most of us already have developed ways of counteracting old not-good-enough stories about ourselves. Basically, when we feel bad, we tend to put ourselves in situations that can be counted on to improve our moods and our self-images. But because big J interferes with these strategies, it has to be blocked—put out of commission itself—before we can tap into our usual feel-good strategies.

The way to resist the J-trance is to remember a time in the past when we did just that. In other words, we have to be able to recall an episode when we were jealous *and* self-assured, a time when, feeling displaced, we nevertheless managed to soothe ourselves. Since few of us have managed to accomplish such an unlikely feat, it may be tricky to draw on such a memory. The fact is, we may just have to create one. Fortunately, our new downsized gallery of jealousies makes it possible.

Jealousy for Beginners

There are big Js, little Js, and in-between Js. There are rough Js, smooth Js, sideways Js, and second cousins twice removed of J. Perhaps we see that a four-legged rival provokes us to insane frenzies. In contrast, two-legged rivals only ruffle us slightly. Or perhaps we are nonchalant at the prospect of both quadra- or biped competitors, but when a partner's wit and grace lands her in the limelight at a party, we skulk away and, hidden behind the giant turkey at the buffet, brood about our lack of charisma.

Each set of circumstances is different, and each evokes a different response. Even the most threatening kinds of jealousies—the sexual kind—aren't uniform or one-dimensional. They can be quick stabs or chronic conditions, can leave one twisting in the wind or dodging the phantoms of the past.

All these small Js make jealousy practice a cinch. We simply have to notice next time we find ourselves in a slightly alarming situation. Instead of trying to escape the tiny swarm of self-doubts when our partner is inattentive or

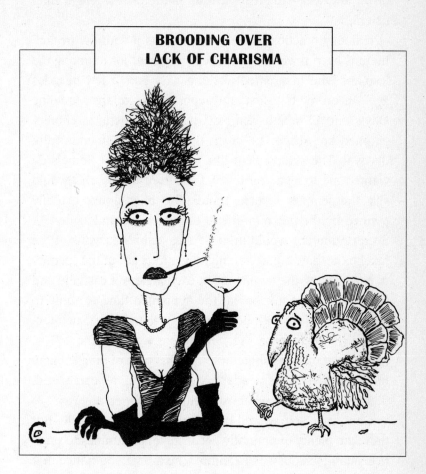

preoccupied with someone else, we simply have to hunker down and wait—to steep in it a minute or two longer than usual.

Jealousy practice is not as strange as it sounds. In fact, there is even a well-documented precedent for it among the lesbians who frequented working-class bars a few decades ago. According to a firsthand report by historians Madeline Davis and Elizabeth Kennedy, butches sometimes choreo-graphed bar scenes in which their femme girlfriends were disloyal. The setups went like this: Mumbling, "Somebody wanted me to give you this," a friend of the butch's would slip the femme a secret note. The billet-doux, actually penned by the butch girlfriend of the femme and signed "A Secret Admirer," would propose a casual rendezvous at the jukebox at, say, 10:30 that night. Curious about the identity of her admirer, the femme might excuse herself casually and sidle over to the jukebox at the appointed time . . . only to come face-to-face with her furiously jealous mate. Such tac-tics might seem crazy. Yet, in the bar world of the 1950s, where relationships shifted rapidly, this type of practice may have been extremely adaptive—a way to rehearse and, thereby, prepare for what was bound to happen anyway.

Obviously, setting well-baited traps is not advisable. But there are plenty of naturally occurring opportunities to prac-tice small-j jealousy. For example, next time you notice that your partner's party conversation with an attractive stranger seems a little too animated, try hesitating an extra minute or two before bustling across the room and collaring her. Or refrain from cross-examining her as zealously as you might ordinarily when she comes home from a dinner with an ex-flame. Notice how easy it is to hit high C of anxiety or slide down the intensity scale, to minimize or maximize the amount of tolerable queasiness.

After you've gotten the hang of these small jealousies, you might even want to practice a couple of more advanced Js. Try spending part of an evening apart without reporting on your activities.

Let's say the worst-case scenario happens. Your girlfriend comes back and informs you she's had a fling. You get the jitters: you sweat, pace, cry, get pissed. And here's the surprise. You have already crafted your new story without even knowing it. During your practice sessions, you already changed the old jealousy story about being powerless. You already knew how to be cool, collected, and jealous. As it turns out, the latest development isn't all that big a deal. A little more intense, but not all that different. In fact, you tell her—after punishing her sufficiently—it's okay this time, but just don't let it happen again or you'll get your cousin Mario to break little whatshername's kneecaps.

After that episode, you put the finishing touches on your new J-proof story. It isn't an epic where an unlikely hero whups a Goliath jealousy. Instead, you now have a humble tale about survival after a brush with a junior J in your repertoire. Despite its modest scope, it has done the trick. You can now draw on a memory of jealousy competency.

Big J may come again. Your temples may pound with the same ferocity. You may be mad with misery. Still, you'll never be able to be hypnotized as you once were. No matter how bad it gets.

Chapter 7

Turning Down the Jezebel Decibels

There is another tale or two that we might want to add to our small but growing antijealousy kit. Instead of featuring our own modest triumphs, these other stories showcase an even more improbable heroine: the other woman.

One of the main imports from the het culture is a folk myth about mate stealers: those designing and unscrupulous females who break up happy couples. According to the myth, these sorcerers work their wiles on unsuspecting partners, luring them away from the hearths and hearts that hold them dear. We might call these tales "jealousy-feeder myths." Big-J jealousy depends on them. If we hadn't been thoroughly steeped in such tall tales, that green-eyed monster might lose its clout—might even become a diminutive creature cute enough to cuddle.

The best way to get rid of the feeder stories that nourish jealousy is to replace them with different sorts of other-woman fables. Instead of cautionary tales that feature scheming couple busters, these rehabilitated other women can be harmless diversions or valuable fantasies. In some cases, they can even enhance our relationships.

Positive Other-Woman Stories

The following tales are only the beginning of myriad possibilities. Positive other-women stories are all around us. As soon as we turn down the Jezebel decibels, we will begin to hear them.

The Other Woman as Occasional Lark

RAND, VICTORIA, AND VICTORIA'S SECRET

The workshop was such a groaner that even though they had never met, the two of them were immediately joined in a communion of horrified eye rolling. Without any prearranged signal, they both escaped before the question-and-answer period. Once in the hallway, they decided to draft a protest letter to the conference chair about the ineptness of the presenter. But instead, they just had coffee and talked. After an hour together, spending the night together was a foregone conclusion.

The next day, when Victoria caught her flight home, she decided not to tell her partner what had happened. But somehow Rand knew. When she insisted that Victoria smelled different, Victoria blurted out, "But I took a shower."

"A shower after what?" Rand asked acidly. And Victoria confessed. It was nothing, she assured Rand. She had no intention of seeing her again.

The never-to-be-repeated slip at a conference or a weekend away may be a story that we've heard and dismissed with a shrug. But instead of forgetting the story or filing it away under "Ho hum," we might want to retrieve it, consider it carefully—even give it a more reputable role in our stock of other-women stories. Why? In the first place, the partner who has been dallying may be wrestling with another megamyth. Because she had a great time, she may be telling herself such a chance encounter was a one-in-a-million long shot. How can she ignore such an obvious subpoena from Cupid? She would be a fool not to follow up—not to seize such an opportunity. And an encore would be so easy to arrange. A few keystrokes, and thousands of miles dissolve instantly.

For most of us, the line between meaningful and casual is a fine one. Just how fine is evident in the account of lesbians who have sex outside the contexts of dating or long-term relationships. Robin, a friend and frequenter of Bay Area lesbian sex clubs, recalls a recent encounter at the Ecstasy Lounge: "We had a wonderful time ... tender, caring, exciting. Afterward, we talked for a while and showered. I made sure to get her address and phone number. For the next couple of weeks, I played with the idea of calling or writing. Then I got a note from her: she had been wondering whether to call me. She wasn't sure if she would, but she told me she had a wonderful time and gave me her address and phone number again. I sent a similar note back to her. Neither of us ever called."

As both women contemplated making something more of their encounter, their future hung in the air. But perhaps because both were experienced one-timers, they decided not to pursue it. Robin's summary: "It was a delightful memory . . . one of the most pure, definable relationships I ever had."

While such brief encounters foreclose one kind of future, they open a door on another one—that is, the permanent possibility of such miniaturized relationships. Part art form, part serendipity, one-time meetings offer us a gift. But in order to accept it, we have to have a readily available story that tells us that these experiences can be both exquisite and complete. Being able to tell such a meaningful ministory is vital for the partner who has had a fling. And it is equally important for her primary partner. Why?

Because, contrary to popular opinion, the glue that holds couples together is not sex or good communication. It is mutual storytelling. The more couples can improvise together as they go along—weave events into collaborative stories—the sturdier their relationships will be. Take the example of the conference fling. Say the partner of the one-timer knows only two-timing stories. What if, as soon as she

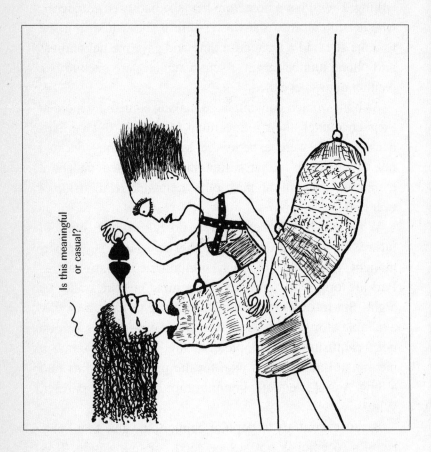

hears what happened at the conference, she starts invoking the standard other-woman doomsday scenario? All hopes of any collaboration are dashed. In reaction, her wavering partner is likely to become defensive and guilty. Eager to find some credibility for *her* story, she is much more likely to look for confirmation from the only other person who knows the encounter was casual. She calls her conference buddy, only to find out that she also got a hostile reception at home. Now the two have much more reason for bonding than their brief fling provided: they can commiserate about their intolerant lovers. It is this collaboration rather than anything erotic that forms the basis of their new relationship.

On the other hand, if the stay-at-home partner has her own well-developed fund of girlz-will-be-boyz capers (and has done her jealousy practice), she may even embellish her partner's fling story with a few lewd observations or recollections of her own indiscretions. The result: by converting a potentially divisive tale into a whimsical fable, the couple have proven that their partnership is strong enough to withstand outside sex.

Perhaps next time they go out with friends, they may even jointly relate the story to the rapt group: "As soon as she came off the plane, I knew. I could smell it." "Yeah," her partner retorts with a mock scowl, "she always told me about the summer her mother bred bloodhounds. Before this, I always thought she just meant her mother *raised* them." Their friends' amused reactions to the story further certifies the sturdiness of the couple.

The Modular Other Woman

Impetuous-moment stories are important additions to every couple's jealousy prevention kit. Another kind of story installs the other woman more permanently in the life of the couple. Harder to tell, these stories are nevertheless an equally important addition to anti-J repertoires.

SIRI AND RUSTY

When Siri, a starry-eyed twenty-five-year-old, first arrived in San Francisco, she made a beeline for gay bars and found herself in the middle of Carnival. Ms. and Mr. Leather were in the process of being crowned at a popular hot spot. In the ensuing revelry, Siri went home with a runner-up. By the next morning, she and Rusty were an item.

From the beginning, part of the Rusty package was a Saturday night play party once or twice a month. The rest of the time, the two of them were indistinguishable— except perhaps for an occasional private scene—from the vanilla couple next-door. A year later, Siri and Rusty broke up. When Siri started seeing someone new, she was surprised to find out that Saturday night parties were not automatically part of dating. And even more amazed to realize that her new girlfriend expected a sexually exclusive relationship.

In 1951, anthropologists Clellan Ford and Frank Beach published the first exhaustive study of sexual practices around the globe. The two researchers found 17 out of 139 societies in which extramarital relations were extremely common. Probably they were not even counting a unique cluster of lesbians. Along with the Chukchee of Siberia, the Ammassalik of Greenland, and the Banaro of New Guinea, a small band of lesbians has learned to tell their own unique other-woman stories. Under certain circumstances, both partners assume the other woman exists. From time to time, one or both partners will have sex with her.

How is it possible for couples to tell tales that run so counter to most other-woman stories? These gifted story-tellers start with an entirely different premise: instead of expecting lifelong fidelity, these partners believe it is only a matter of time until the potentially disruptive outsider shows up on their doorstep. They don't wait for their hunch to materialize. Applying a strategy that sociologists call "anticipatory coping," they prepare for the inevitable knock on the door by putting up a series of greeting signs: Yo, stranger! Welcome! We've been expecting you. No, don't enter here. Go around the corner. Take the second door to the left, and follow the green arrow. You'll find a small but well-appointed room at the end of the corridor. Make yourself comfortable.

In other words, certain partners define the separate quarters of the newcomer in terms of a series of dos and don'ts. For example, one couple may agree that playing at sex parties or clubs is okay, but private dates are off-limits. Other lesbian couples establish different ways to encapsulate the other woman. Outside dates, for example, are permitted, but they can occur only, say, on Wednesday nights. As long as she is securely contained, the other woman can become a staple, even a relationship enhancer—as predictable and indispensable as a regular yearly vacation. A few mutually agreed-upon rules can turn potentially menacing intruders into insignificant others.

The Invisible Other Woman

Another way to neutralize the other-woman threat is to enlarge each partner's personal sphere. After a slight adjustment in what each partner accepts as a "normal" amount of privacy, cheating is no longer possible. The tired old tale of the secret affair becomes a story of healthy boundary maintenance.

MARGOT AND RISH

Margot and Rish refer to themselves as space queens. But they didn't start out that way. Five years ago, just when they were about to move in together, an old girlfriend of Rish's resurfaced. According to Margot and Rish, if they had been under the same roof at the time, they wouldn't have weathered the affair. As it was, they barely spoke for a year after it was over. But Rish persevered in making amends, and eventually Margot relented. Or rather, she adopted a wait-and-see policy.

During the probation period, both came to realize that there would be other problems if they lived together. Margot requires a certain amount of squalor to function, whereas Rish is a neat freak. Rish uses Mozart for background noise, and Margot never turns off the sports channel. So they decided to make their temporary living-apart status permanent. Now, each suits herself when she is alone.

Having learned the hard way that they can't survive outside affairs, they have decided to limit information about them. They spend most nights together, at one apartment or the other; but for one day and night, each week, they have agreed to log off each other's gaydar screens. As far as each is concerned, the other could be watching football, picking lint off the carpet, or having orgies. Mostly, they confide confidentially, they spend the time wishing they could be together.

When partners first get together, they may have different ideas about what is mine, yours, and ours. Time, money, even how many daydreams to share are up for discussion. And no two relationships are alike. For some couples, the "us" pile is so huge it dwarfs both the "me" and "her" stacks. In less mutually oriented partnerships, the opposite may be true. And, of course, the stacks aren't static. Renegotiations are always under way. In a given week, for example, one partner may want more together time, the other more alone time. Or, if they move in together, they may decide to pool resources to pay for household expenses. As a result, the togetherness pile may surge.

Acknowledged or not, many couples also have three sex stacks. There is ours, yours, and my sex. Private sex may consist of a favorite fantasy or a vibrator quickie after a girlfriend has gone to work. The erotic activities in one's private domain are not exactly secret. But just as we don't divulge the amount we paid for a pair of birthday earrings, we don't announce every time we plug in Magic Wanda.

In other words, the ongoing collaborative story that most partners tell about their relationships includes a chapter or two about privacy. In most cases, this privacy does not extend to other sexual partners. Yet, what if it did? What if, right between the chapters entitled "Time Apart" and "Separate Friendships," there were a section called "Private Part(ner)s?"

Because there is a cultural consensus about certain kinds of privacies, most couples don't even have to agree about rules. We take it for granted, for example, that we won't listen in on our partner's phone conversations or open her mail. The fact that there is a great hullabaloo when such violations do occur only proves that a partner has, indeed, stepped over the line.

When it comes to other women, however, an opposite set of unstated cultural rules immediately goes into effect. As mates, we *know* we must be vigilant—head off any Jezebel headed our way. Therefore, previously taboo behavior—spying, prying, or even hiring private detectives—is suddenly culturally mandated. If either partner suspects an other-woman invasion, she is almost obligated to violate her partner's privacy in ways she would never consider under any other circumstances.

In order to tell new stories, therefore, we needn't find ways to domesticate or diminish the other woman. We need only consciously extend the usual cultural rules about privacy—the ones that already apply to our fantasies and our vibrator—to other sexual partners. How? There are plenty of ways to tell the Private Part(ner)s story.

For example, some partners agree to being unaccountable to each other during certain specified periods of time. During the blackouts, each is free to do what she likes without reporting in. By mutual consent, all traces of other partners are meticulously removed from housing and conversation.

Still other partners may prefer the information filter to be partial. In other words, they prefer to know about the existence of other sexual partners but want to be spared all the details.

For example, after much discussion about what each needed to know about her partner's extramarital encounters, one couple devised a postsex questionnaire that included the following multiple choice queries:

1. If your fling had placed a personals ad, what would it say? (e.g., "married babe seeks chick on the side").

2. How would you rate this experience?
   It sucked
   Not sure if it was worth it
   It was better than sitting at home
   It was as good as *Red Rock West*
   It blew my mind
   It changed my life
   Jury is not in yet

3. How would you rate this person overall?
> Serial killer
> Drip
> Unremarkable
> Nice
> Really cool
> Want this person in my life (sexual interest dead)
> Can imagine long-term something (my interest isn't dead)
> Can imagine falling in love (my interest isn't dead)

4. Should I worry about the state of our relationship?
> No, you should join me in laughing at this pathetic person who tried to pursue me.
> No, you should be happy that I'm having fun and learning new tricks.
> You should know that this person is important to me and I plan to have her in my life in some way.
> Yes. A letter follows.

Another couple consciously made information about outside sex optional. Each kept a brief log of her encounters with other women. Both partners' record books, which listed only names, places, and dates, were left on top of the bookcase—available for either to check if she so desired. One partner never checked the log. After a peek or two, the other stopped.

This kind of other-woman story can be told in many ways. Even so, it may not suit all storytellers. For example, the inadvertent clairvoyants among us may be at a distinct disadvantage. Intentional informational blackouts don't work for those of us who rely on ESP to track our partner's moods and maneuverings. In fact, for the very sensitive, maintaining the psychological space required for private part(ner)s may not be possible under the same roof. And living apart may not be a desirable option. For many couples, the delights of living together clearly outweigh the more uncertain pleasures of privacy.

One couple, however, seems to have devised an eat-your-cake-and-have-it-too solution. Eager to maintain a high level of privacy *and* intimacy—and avoid the schlep factor of cross-town apartments—the women live in separate flats in the same building. Together for ten years, they seem to have proved that forever-after is indeed a multistoreyed affair.

When they need privacy in small quarters, the Japanese use shoji screens to cordon off certain areas. These room dividers can be shifted according to the needs of the moment: a child's play area in the morning becomes a dining room in the evening and a bedroom at night. It doesn't take a heavy weight to move the light-as-a-feather shoji screens. A subtle touch will do it. And even though the illusion is transparent, it gets the job done. If we figure out ways to devise our own shoji screens, we are relieved of the necessity of telling any stories at all about the other woman.

The Other Woman as Permanent Partner

Another set of lesbians, perhaps the wily coyotes of the dyke tribe, also balk at other-woman stories, negative *or* positive. Their solution to the problem? They simply turn the outsider into an insider. They marry the other woman.

PJ, KELSEN, AND DANA

Longtime political activists and permanent partners, PJ and Kelsen were PFLAG darlings, the twosome who could be counted on to showcase their relationship whenever any lesbian or gay organization needed to display a lesbian poster couple. They got to know Dana when she joined the board of the AIDS hospice. Over the next year, all three had ample opportunity to work together on fundraisers and staffing crises. It seemed only natural when Dana broke up with her girlfriend for Kelsen and PJ to offer her their spare bedroom. And even more natural, after about six months, to invite her into their bed. That was six years ago. Since then, they've bought a new king-sized bed and a house big enough to accommodate it.

Mention threesomes, and most of us conjure up the relationship-from-hell story. In a desperate effort to ward off a me-or-her ultimatum—a forced choice between a new and old lover—both members of the couple agree to an experiment. Somehow they will find a way to include the newcomer in their partnership. The ensuing folie à trois is foreshadowed in the first stanzas of "Field," a poem by lesbian poet Olga Broumas:

I had a lover. Let us say we were married, owned
a house, shared a car. . . .

In time, my lover came to take
another lover, of whom I also became enamored.
There is a seagull floating backward in a rare

snowstorm on an Atlantic Ocean bay as I remember this,
its head at an angle that suggests amusement.

Had they been as detached as the bird, the poem makes clear, they might have avoided a tempestuous free-for-all. But, despite Broumas's bittersweet reflections, third parties are just what some couples need. In certain cases, the incorporation of the other woman into seasoned relationships can stabilize, and even enhance, partnerships.

When an old friend told me she had met a long-term threesome, I asked her to introduce me. Next time I visited her in Albuquerque, she arranged for me to meet them. Over the next six months, the Internet helped me find and interview two other long-term threesomes.

A dozen hours spent with three threesomes hardly constitutes an in-depth study of such relationships. But it does suggest that under certain circumstances, long-term partners can and do successfully reconfigure their twosomes into permanent threesomes. How and why do such arrangements develop?

Actually, if we think about it for a minute, it becomes evident that threesomes are not exceptional. No matter how coupled we are, we rarely remain in actual twosomes for very long. Our intimacies are not hermetically sealed. Typically, pets or parents, children or friends are constantly joining and expanding our magic circle. In fact, most of us probably spend more time in threesomes and foursomes than we do in twosomes.

Sometimes the newcomer's presence is disruptive. Or sometimes the addition becomes a fulcrum, correcting a dangerous wobble between the two partners. Because these third parties aren't dreaded other women, however, we hardly notice the frequency of their comings and goings.

Each of the three threesomes I interviewed had evolved in a different fashion. One of the long-term arrangements was inaugurated when both members of a couple became simultaneously attracted to someone new and agreed to invite her aboard. In another situation, the already convinced—and smitten—half of the couple acted as Cupid between her dubious partner and the new recruit. In the third, one of the original partners was significantly older than her longtime partner. Because she was no longer interested in sex, she suggested that her partner find another sexual partner. Her partner obliged.

One of the threesomes had only three-way sex. Another alternated between two- and threesomes. In the third, where the sexually disinterested partner participated in the threesome in primarily nonsexual ways, only two of the partners were erotically linked.

Whether or not such relationships should be "open" to new members was just as much of a sticking point as it is for most twosomes. One threesome closed ranks quickly, declaring themselves sexually exclusive. Another, opting for a yeastier brew, continued to look for new family members. The third, like many twosomes, remains divided—and embattled—over the issue of open or closed boundaries.

The partners who made up these trios were very different from one another. In addition to ages that ranged, in one threesome, from thirty-one to seventy-two, partners had different backgrounds and occupations. The Albuquerque partnership, for example, consisted of a forty-year-old Hispanic pilot, a forty-two-year-old Jewish house painter, and a twenty-eight-year-old WASP who worked for minimum wage in a nonprofit agency (and who had changed her name in order not to embarrass her conservative Republican parents).

What struck me about all three partnerships was what I might call resource intensiveness. When we think of threesomes, the metaphor of the third wheel—the unwanted extra—immediately comes to mind. After my exposure to these trios, however, the old metaphor never quite recovered its former potency. On the contrary, the extra wheel was usually an asset. Whenever a particular need arose, somebody was on hand to take care of it. For example, if someone was short of cash that week, someone else pitched in to cover household expenses. Ditto for emotional support, sexual energy, child care help, even companionship.

All this extra resourcefulness didn't come without a price. The profusion of people, pets—and in one household, two children plus a gang of their chums—probably made a quiet evening at home unlikely. And, besides being part of these abundant households, each of the women had her own outside life—friends, work, and recreational activities. Consequently, the appointment books of the partners resembled the radar screens in the traffic control tower at JFK. In fact, in order to manage the volume of incoming and outgoing messages, one of the three households boasted three phone lines, three computers, and two faxes.

In addition to the necessity for all the outside world links, the trios required more time for discussion about everything from hurt feelings to chores. Agreements about how to minimize friction among these ménages had to be painstakingly hammered out. Item number nine in one of the threesomes' twenty-page contract, for example, reads as follows: "Household currently owns and maintains three cats and three dogs. Additional family pets or pets replacing existing animals which would impact family finances or shared spaces must be approved by all co-owners. If, however, an individual wishes to have a new pet which will reside exclusively in its mistress' office (e.g., fish or a caged pet), consensus is not required."

Diverse and lively as these arrangements were, there was one thing all the threesomes had in common. Though each woman was open about her lesbianism, all were very discreet about their current arrangements. Outside of a few trusted friends or close family members, no one knew about their three-way intimacies. It's not surprising. Lesbian couples are still on the fringes of reputability. What chance is there that a trio of loving women would be viewed with anything other than suspicion and hostility? Consequently, these trios have more than one reason for their extralarge closets. Unfortunately, their necessary protective secrecy shortchanges us all. As a result, most of us will never have a chance to be directly exposed to a truly unique other-woman story.

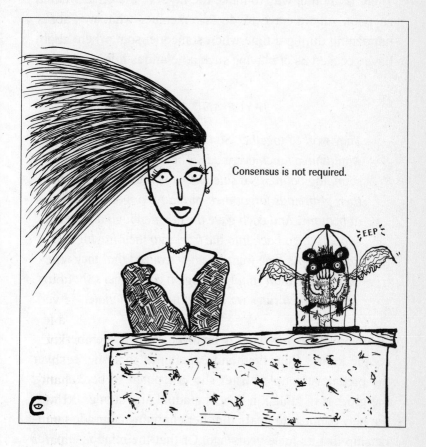

The Inner Other Woman

There is another way to make the myth of the other woman go poof. All we have to do is remember what was really happening during a time when someone, somewhere might have accused us of playing such a nefarious role.

JAYCE AND KIM

They worked together. So it was only natural that they would have lunch every day. They used the other as a sounding board, as a safe place to grouse, to vent when their girlfriends forgot their birthdays or got headaches at bedtime. And each gave the other enough advice and support to go back into the fray, into their fraying relationships. As time went by, they realized that they were doing more than simply crying on each other's shoulders and that their hugs were more than affectionate.

Anyone who has gotten involved with a member of a couple knows from firsthand experience that she is never the predatory couple buster she is reputed to be. Usually, the process of falling in love is gradual and subtle. Perhaps the new confidante hears that her charming comrade's partnership lost its juice years ago. Or that the relationship, far from moribund, is excruciatingly alive—a source of conflict and pain for both partners. Even, however, in cases where the budding relationship between the two new friends is the catalyst for the breakup of an old relationship, the other woman probably feels ill at ease, torn, guilty.

The malevolent home wrecker is a cartoon character. And there is nothing like firsthand experience to help us see through the stereotype. But some lesbians choose to take the caricature one step further. They purposefully assume the other-woman label.

Lesbians are expert epithet-recyclers. We regularly refashion frequently hurled insults—"dyke" and "queer," for example—into proudly worn badges of honor. A few talented reclamation artists among us have worked similar magic on the negative stereotype of the other woman. Not only have they reclaimed the label, but also they have put a positive spin on it. Instead of vultures who prey upon vulnerable relationships, these "other women" view themselves as guardian angels of couples, the saviors who rescue long-term partnerships from the dangerous shoals of ennui.

Mostly it starts as a joke. Women who are involved with half of a couple start referring jocularly to themselves as the other woman. And then, after observing their patterns over time, they get more earnest about the role.

Lesbians who claim that they make an erotic and emotional career out of being other women usually find their niche after discovering—often the hard way—that being coupled simply doesn't suit them. For example, one self-identified other woman sorts her relationships into three types. The first are casual, one-night stands. The second type, long-term partnerships, have consistently felt limited and limiting to her. The third kind of relationship—those in which she is involved over time with one or both members of a couple—have been her most nurturing and sustaining attachments.

Another lesbian who characterizes herself as the other woman has ongoing relationships with two women, each of whom is in an open, long-term permanent partnership. Neither has any intention of leaving their partners for her, and she has no desire to run off into the sunset with either of them.

These other women claim they make a significant contribution to coupledom. They are providing primary intimates with a safe diversion. Because of the presence of these other women in their lives, long-term partners can experience the excitement no longer available in their secure relationships. And, in return, the other woman gets what she is craving: Never taken for granted, she can be on permanent honeymoon. Nor does she have to report to anyone about her comings and goings. Never in danger of being enmeshed in a twosome, she can be lighthearted about multiple relationships. Despite the rules they had set up in previous primary relationships, until now such a guilt-free state, they claim, had always eluded them.

When we have opportunities to tell our own original other-woman stories, the caricature of the master manipulator dissolves. Instead, the other woman, caught up in currents of change that are impossible to resist, may be tormented herself. Or perhaps she is a free spirit, someone whose much-desired independence meshes nicely with certain long-term partners' desire for outside diversions. More like ecologists than home wreckers, these other women can have the same beneficial effect on long-term partnerships as controlled burns do on the maintenance of healthy forests.

The Other Woman as Forever-After Partner

Even without a face or a form, the other woman can be our ally. She can be a vital remembrance of things past, or a bridge to the future. She can be a foil for our living, breathing relationship or a crystal ball that reveals all sorts of otherwise inaccessible secrets.

BARB AND MAGGIE

It was a funny thing. After a decade together, it became clear to Barb that Maggie wasn't going to leave her for someone else. The other woman whom Barb had always feared had never materialized. It was at that point that the sea change happened. Barb's fantasy tilted wildly and made a 180-degree turn. Instead of a marauder who would steal Maggie, the other woman she had been so afraid of turned into her own phantom lover. Vague, yet enticing, she was more a possibility than a person. She was an inviting envoy from the world beyond their relationship.

At first, the notion of intentionally dreaming up the other woman sounds as preposterous as having a piranha for a pet. But not if we think about it for a moment. Our lives teem with phantoms. These apparitions—typically in the form of abusive or simply absent parents—have a tendency to rattle their skeletons just when we thought we were safe at last. Or, instead of the ghosts of parents, they are ex-lovers we would just as soon forget. Just when we are getting ready to curl up with our girlfriends, they do a wild fandango across the bedroom.

Many of us spend small fortunes in time and energy and money trying to exorcise these phantoms. But instead of trying to dislodge our virtual visitors, why not add a benign spirit guide or two to our mental menageries? One who might exert a more positive influence?

Such additions to our spirit families are particularly important for those of us who specialize in the souls of others. Plenty of us work at jobs that require great amounts of hand-holding. Others of us, conscientious mothers and dutiful daughters and accommodating partners, simply nurture out of love or habit. Paid or unpaid, full-time caretakers rarely have time to reflect on the state of their own souls. Preoccupied with the needs of others, usually such mind readers *extraordinaire* have not cultivated the habit of probing their own psyches. Here's where the other woman comes in. When we conjure up our heart's desire, we create a delicate mirroring device. Other-women fantasies are crystal balls that reveal our souls.

Try for just a minute to summon her up. Perhaps she never quite comes into focus. Instead she is a vague longing for what might be—a nameless, faceless melancholy. About what? About everything and nothing. About life.

Or perhaps her contours are faintly familiar. Perhaps though not exactly a replica of someone who was once important to us, the new fantasy has the qualities of an ex. Perhaps, in our determination to put the past behind us, we have overlooked the fact that—along with all her disagreeable traits—there are qualities in an ex-partner that we miss and long for.

In other words, who we conjure up tells us something about what we are missing. If someone unfamiliar swims into view, be sure to examine her closely. Notice her hair, the way she walks, her breasts, her clothes. Is she older or younger? Bigger or smaller? Darker or lighter? All these details will tell us something about the state of our souls. If she turns out to be a Christiane Annapour clone who shuttles between Beirut and Sarajevo on assignments for CNN, chances are we are missing a certain on-the-edge-frisson. If she is a Jody Foster look-alike, whom we sport on our arm, chances are we are limelight deprived. If an earth mother smothers us in bosomy hugs, we might be feeling undernurtured.

You might want to develop your other-woman fantasy. Install her as your permanent muse. Pay attention to her. She'll tell you whether to sign up for a scuba class or just buy some new lingerie. And after you do what she suggests, check in with her from time to time. Has she changed? Is she suggesting another direction? You are entitled to keep her to yourself. She is, after all, purely your playmate, soul mate—combination projection, reflection, guide. And, Aphrodite forbid, if anything should ever happen to your partner, your fantasy lover will be there for you. She will share your memories and your tears. She will console and commiserate. And, one day, when the time is right, she will lead you back to the world.

Welcome to the Global Gay Village

An ample supply of positive other-women anecdotes is not a magic pill. Such stories will not prevent suspicion or cure a breaking heart. They will never curb old familiar nightmares or incite a glorious revolution in intimacy. On the other hand, these stories may give our relationships the extra durability necessary to weather the ticklish situations that are likely to come up during the course of our relationships.

"We are everywhere" is a wonderfully affirming statement when it applies to all those institutions previously off-limits. The more lesbians and gays who manage to infiltrate the military, hold public office, or crack the lavender ceiling inside a Fortune 500 corporation, the better. But what about our private lives? Do we really want so many queers around after we have found our mate? When our lover has lunch with cruisy coworkers every day or has cozy electronic chats with intriguing strangers every night, we may feel like "we are everywhere" is just a keystroke away from "I am nowhere."

Hooked up and hypermobile, plenty of us now interface with dykes more often than we go to the bathroom. The sheer volume of queer contact almost guarantees that even after we have found our true love and settled down, we will probably experience flashpoints—hot connections that, in the best of all possible worlds, would be reserved for lovers.

The stories we tell shape our lives. If we have only one story about forever-after, a tale about cloistered twosomes who always renounce the world's temptations, these inevitable flameups along the way are much likely to turn our partnerships into flameouts. At the first knock on the cloister door, we will be convinced that our worst fears have come true. We know it. We can feel it in our bones: Our darling is in the process of leaving us. It is only a matter of time. Or, just as terrifying, we are the ones abandoning our mates. And the pain or guilt about such perceived betrayal may even hasten the end.

Paradoxically, the effect of the forever-after story can be even more damaging in situations where partnerships don't dissolve. Let's say, upon hearing news that an attractive stranger is lurking nearby, we beef up the border patrols. Nobody is going anywhere, we vow through gritted teeth. Even if our determination heads off a break-in or breakup, the price of forever-after may be high, too high. Ensconced in our newly reinforced, us-against-them fortresses, we are likely to feel more besieged than beloved.

But what if we have other stories in our repertoire? Instead of limiting ourselves to fables about hermetically sealed relationships, we might have plenty of other tales about the periodic comings and goings of strangers. The visitors might be irresistible waifs who remind us of the blessings we have been taking for granted. Or envoys who bring enchanting news of faraway places we never even suspected existed. Perhaps our mi-casa-su-casa hospitality knows no bounds. Then again, it might be limited to a single night . . . at the crack of dawn, the guests must move on.

Stories about the myriad ways in which other women can make valuable contributions to our lives won't render our relationships intruder proof. Nothing can do that. But, in today's meet-market world, such tales will make our partnerships safer.

Chapter 8

Private Rituals, Public Ceremonies: How We Tell Our Stories

When I want to scandalize my urbane friends, I announce I am thinking of joining a coven. "Surely," they huff and puff, "you can't be serious! You can't believe in all that hocus-pocus!" As we debate the pros and cons of women's spirituality, I gradually inch my way over to their bulletin boards and start fiddling with their meticulously placed objects. Or else I sidle over to their desks and begin to riffle through a stack of papers. The resultant howls of protest prove that even dyed-in-the-wool secularists have their own altars and amulets. They simply call them by different names. With the sites of their secret rites exposed, they may concede I have a point.

"But what about spell casting?" they inquire dubiously. Surely I don't believe that burning incense and calling on the Goddess can help a budding romance? Then I remind these unconscious *curanderas* of their own magic making— the times I have sat and watched them prepare for their own dates by, systematically and methodically, trying on every T-shirt and every pair of jeans in their wardrobes.

Whether we subscribe to the world according to Levi Strauss or Z Budapest, we need our rituals. They are the way we counteract another story, the ubiquitous tale told by means of silence—or worse, by changed subjects and averted eyes. When we don denim or light candles or add a particularly piquant Alison Bechdel cartoon to our bulletin boards, we are refusing to collaborate with the erasure of our lives and loves. Instead, rituals offer us a way of turning up the volume on our own stories.

There is one dyke ritual so compelling that even my most bah-humbug friends mingle contentedly with their less worldly sisters. Secularists and spiritualists alike seem to love lesbian commitment ceremonies. Why? Not just because of the food (though it is always sublime) or the multicultural exuberance (where else can you find two brides standing under a chuppah designed by Hopis or hear Gershwin on gamelan?). Rather, the appeal of these rituals comes from their ability to silence the other story. For a few hours the ceaseless din that bombards us on airplanes and buses and freeways, on NBC and CBS, in movies and books, at home and at work is silenced by the performance of our own quirky and giddy romances.

For those of us who have been witness starved for so long, the most thrilling part of the ceremony is the presence of friendly outsiders. We sneak peeks or gawk openly at Aunt Ida and Uncle Harry, at cousins Louise and Delphine, at Shirley and Stanley and Arthur and Myrtle. Even though the gaggle of relatives may have preferred another love story, they are moved to tears by this one. As for those of us witnessing the witnesses, we don't know whether to laugh out loud or cry from sheer joy.

Unfortunately, our stories are not loud enough or long enough to silence that other discounting story for very long. And, as soon as our ceremonies are over, it begins again—even more relentlessly than before.

One couple arrived home after the ceremony to find the teenaged son of one watching football. "But," sputtered his mother, "this was such an important day to me. You promised you'd be there!"

"Jeez, Mom, get a clue," he replied without taking his eyes off the TV. "You can't marry a girl."

Another couple, off on their honeymoon in Maui, elected to take a "lovebird" boat tour of a famous grotto. The boat was packed with het couples, all holding hands. The lesbian lovers dared not demonstrate any affection and, in addition, had to continually deflect the usual "Are-you-two-girls-here-alone?" questions. As the "Hawaiian Wedding Song" was piped into the grotto, the tour guide told a romantic story about a pair of star-crossed lovers who had perished there. The guide exhorted the honeymooners to make a wish (guaranteed to come true because of the hovering spirits of the departed lovers) and seal it with a kiss. When they could be sure no one was watching, the lesbian newlyweds squeezed each other's hands.

Yet another pair of newlyweds was amazed to discover that even though both sets of parents had come to their ceremony, neither would put up a photograph of the couple in their homes. However, the wedding pictures of all their heterosexual siblings were prominently displayed.

The power of the other story is never more apparent than when we dare give ourselves over entirely to the telling of our own. Yet, in spite of the postceremony shock so commonly reported, few of us regret proclaiming our love publicly. In fact, the pleasurable memories of the ceremony can surface even after the union has dissolved.

"You'd think I wouldn't want to think about it," a recently separated lesbian client tells me. "Just shove the memories, the pictures in the closet. But I don't. It was such a positive experience. I don't have words to explain why it means so much to me, even now."

Because of the surrounding silences, telling the story of our unions is vital to us. In order to recruit a rapt audience, we don't have to spend thousands of dollars or organize gala events. We simply have to notice the witnesses already at hand. Our lovers are only too glad to hear us tell our stories. Whenever we use an endearment, frame a special photo, bring home a treat, we are performing these tales. In fact, for plenty of couples, once-upon-a-time starts when they wake up in the morning.

The Sun Also Rises: Morning Rituals

The first star of the evening appears. Wish I may, wish I might. The distant shimmer of galaxies always seems to evoke the close-up beating of hearts. Night is the perfect time for romance. Or is it?

In her autobiographical book *Family Silver*, lesbian sociologist Susan Krieger describes the surprising pleasures of morning romance. Before Krieger left for the day her lover, Fran, would ask her to sit close to her and, looking directly into her eyes, would say, "Je t'adore." Then Fran would pull her close, embrace and stroke her. It was the sweetness of these morning interludes that Krieger remembered "when the nights had long since faded."

When I started asking lesbians about their morning rituals, I felt as spelunkers must after worming their way through miles of subterranean passages to suddenly emerge into a grand gallery, its vaulted ceiling glistening with limestone treasures. As it turns out, Krieger is not unusual. For many women, morning intimacies are more delicious than anything that happens after dark. Some of the tales of morning love I heard were as simple as reading the Sunday paper together, as mundane as a morning snuggle. Others were more elaborate.

One couple told me about their daily coffee-and-muffin ritual. One day one partner prepares the modest repast and serves her lover in bed. The next day, they reverse roles. After the off-duty partner has been served, the morning hostess brings her own breakfast to bed. Together, they discuss the day's events: who will sort the laundry, who will stop for groceries after work, who will cook dinner. As they drain their cups, the server is obliged to inquire whether today is the day her partner has decided to cut back on caffeine. The response is always the same: "No, not today, perhaps tomorrow." After the on-duty lover refills both their cups, they usually widen their circle to include *Today Show* talk show hosts Katie Couric and Matt Lauer. Now, the couple's earlier discussion of the day's events is likely to veer off into national, even international, matters. After pondering world trade dilemmas, deforestation in the Amazon, or unrest in Afghanistan, they snuggle briefly and get up to meet the day.

Another couple share their bedroom (but not their bed) with Sasha, the dashing dachshund. When the alarm goes off, they call sweetly to Sasha. Preferring to snooze on, she ignores them. "Sasha, Sasha," they coax gently. Eventually Sasha opens her eyes grudgingly, gives them a baleful look, and stretches. When she has finished this part of her morning yoga, she is ready for more vigorous calisthenics—the great vault onto their bed. After a few tries, she succeeds in getting enough of a pawhold to pull herself up. Then she crawls between them and gives them a good-morning kiss. The ritual complete, they are all ready to begin the day.

Another couple wake up at different times. The late riser, still dishabille, saunters provocatively past the desk where her lover, an accountant who works at home, is barely visible behind the piles of IRS forms. After the strumpet moons her number-crunching girlfriend, the chase begins. Pursued around and around chairs, piles of papers, computers, the slugabed emits squeals of delight and desperation. Finally, apprehended, she is led back to bed. There the partners loll around for twenty minutes or so, reporting dreams and demanding reparations—in the form of kissing and apologetic cooing—for blanket stealing, snoring, or other misdemeanors perpetrated during the night.

Different as all these rituals are, all six women tell me how bereft they feel when for some reason they must forgo these morning routines. Most of us find ways to condense our relationships into playful holograms or elegant pantomimes, small playlets about togetherness that we perform over and over. Just like the favorite bedtime stories we begged for as children, these stories lose none of their appeal even though we know what's coming next. In fact, we love the tales for their familiarity. Because their turns and twists are as familiar to us as a partner's cockeyed grin, we can whisper them to ourselves when all the lights are out, the storytellers gone to bed.

Our Lovers, Our Witnesses

Our lovers are our best witnesses. But at the 1987 mass gay wedding in Washington, it became obvious to me that witnessing a relationship and simply being in one are not always compatible activities.

The first Washington wedding was a rainbow mob of moods and masquerades. Arrayed in their grandmothers' peau de soie, a couple on my left never broke their marathon clinch. The overalls-clad dyke couple next to them held hands primly, while a dominatrix and her minion, in leather and lace, respectively, smirked self-consciously.

A great hush fell upon the throng as the New Age cleric sonorously exhorted us to honor the solemnity of the occasion. "The marriage vows we are about to take are sacred," she intoned. "They represented a mutual commitment of body and soul. Such a commitment means that the old slate has to be wiped clean," she continued. "We must erase the past. We must forgive and forget all that has gone before."

A plaintive query issued from the center of the throng: "Do we *have* to?" A titter ruffled the crowd. Directly in front of me were two women, ashimmer in silk. All during the ceremony they had stared intently into each other's eyes. When the wave of sniggering rippled around them, one twitched but suppressed the impulse to giggle. She was determined to wrest some sacred meaning from this improbable event. Without family or friends to "see" their union, the partners had to exchange vows and witness themselves at the same time. They simply couldn't afford a giggle.

Perhaps as a way of compensating for the lack of witnesses at the previous event, the 1991 Washington wedding planners provided abundant supplies of colored chalk. The newlyweds now had the means to inscribe their love stories on the sacred pavement for all the world to see. Their tributes, typically scrawled inside lavender hearts or pink triangles, were as unique as their relationships:

Karen loves Junebug loves Karen.
Trud and Amy, ten years. Nuff said.
TR & Duffy, three glorious months.
Wendy, Andrea, Tory, Reilly, Chelsea, Garbo, Elliot:
the perfect family unit

Lisa and Cathy, who would have thought it!!!
Deidre + life
Audrey + ♀ ♀ ♀ ♀
Pooh plus ?

As I ambled among hundreds of such displays of concretized love, I was intercepted repeatedly. Thrusting a Kodak or a Minolta into my hands, a couple would ask me to take a photo of them next to their amorous graffiti. After I had taken half a dozen such photos, I remembered how disappointed two friends of mine, a couple, had been because they had to miss out on the event. I etched a heart on the pavement and scratched their names inside it. Then I photographed the Valentine with my own camera. When I got home, I presented them with a framed photo of their private corner of the Washington ceremony. It occupies a place of honor in their living room.

In order to witness our relationships, to really savor them, we may need to step back, to relocate ourselves briefly outside of here and now. During such time-outs, most of us can envision a way to distill our relationships into an art form. Whether we scratch some initials on tarmac or sketch a girlfriend's silhouette or pen a love poem, we are converting the heartbeat of the relationship into a permanent record.

Cyndee, an Internet pal, tells me she and her partner do it with notes. Notes under pillows, on the kitchen counter, in briefcases and lunch bags. These billets-doux can be simple: "It's Friday and I'm loving you." Or, when life's journey has taken a difficult twist, more substantial: "Good morning, my darling. I'll be with you today. May peace and patience prevail in your day, and you can draw upon your inner strength to know and believe you are a good person. You are a special woman. Be kind to yourself. Go gently."

Another couple prefer to tell their story by proxy. Their stand-ins are a Raggedy Ann doll and a worn button-eyed teddy, affectionately known as Threadbear. The last one to leave the house arranges Ann and Threadbear in a semaphore decipherable only to her partner. Perhaps, for example, Threadbear is going down on Ann. Or perhaps both are hanging from the chandelier (strung up by bungie cord on the ceiling light fixture). Or they are wedged in a pair of pantyhose. The proxies' penchant for such antics has, so far, proved inexhaustible.

Keepsakes can also condense our love stories into a permanent and portable form. Esther, a friend, writes me that "my grad school heartthrob and I still talk on the phone every Sunday. In 1986, on the tenth anniversary of our phone conversations, I flew to where she was doing her postdoc. We each pierced one ear (symbolic of the part of our body that is most closely connected to the phone, I guess) and shared one pair of sapphire ear studs. I lost my ear stud on a ship en route to Antarctica, which means I know exactly where it is, as that ship sank two weeks after I got off."

For the auditorially endowed, visual cues may, so to speak, fall on deaf eyes. In order to be really savored, a love story must be strummed or crooned. Still another group of women prefer to sniff their love stories. When a friend was temporarily assigned to a training course at corporate headquarters three states away, her lover made sure a handkerchief doused with her perfume along with a pair of her day-old panties was tucked away in her lover's totebag.

Such bonsaied love tales are bound to charm their intended audience. But perhaps these stories are even more valuable to their creators. Why? In order to decide whether we will celebrate the erotic or the tender or the supportive aspects of our relationship, we must make an inventory of all of them. In the process of storytelling, we become intensive witnesses—savoring not only the features we decide to celebrate, but also all the juicy details on the cutting room floor.

Recruiting Outside Witnesses

Most of us—by necessity—have become adept at telling and listening to our own stories. Yet, in spite of the shortage of outside witnesses, we need not be our only audiences. Recruiting outside witnesses is itself an art form—a gift as important to cultivate as storytelling itself.

A few years ago an anonymous caller left a mysterious message on my machine. She wanted to make an appointment for herself and her lover. But for reasons that would become clear, she couldn't leave a number for me to call her back. She went on to say when she would call back. She hoped I would be in during at least one of those calls and would pick up the phone. When she did finally reach me, she told me that she and her woman lover were taking no chances about anyone blowing their cover. Both were happily married. To men. As far as their husbands and families were concerned, the two women were simply close friends. Because they participated together in so many community activities, no one questioned their schedules or their closeness.

She knew that the therapy relationship was supposed to be confidential, but even so . . . Her voice trailed off. They were both afraid, she continued, of doing anything to jeopardize their relationship. But at the same time, after ten years, it was time to let someone in on their secret. They had no problems. They simply wanted to tell their story to an outsider, someone they could be sure was safely outside of the loop of their families and communities.

Most couples aren't so closeted or so succinct about their reasons for coming to therapy. Yet, when I am puzzled about why partners whose problems seem to have been resolved continue to come to therapy, I think of the clandestine couple. All lesbian couples, closeted or not, are largely invisible. Part of my usefulness as a therapist is being able to provide reflections for couples who have no other mirrors. At times, it may be worthwhile to hire a professional witness; yet there are plenty of other ways to be seen and heard by outsiders.

Mentioning our partners consistently in conversations with family or friends or sending cards signed by both partners are simple methods of recruiting outside witnesses for our relationships. One couple I know traditionally turns a "family" photo into a holiday card. Roped together with Xmas lights or posing on a Hawaiian beach with snorkel gear and Santa hats, the two wish relatives and friends peace on earth and a warm and happy new year.

One openly gay friend shares a large office with six women coworkers. From time to time her lover sends her flowers. The first time, her colleagues gathered around to admire the bouquet. Had she been holding out, they wanted to know. Was it her birthday? She shook her head and passed around the card. Signed by her partner, it read, "Just because I love you."

Afterward whenever she was on the phone with her lover, one of her coworkers would wink lewdly and stage-whisper to everyone else that "just because" was on the phone. Now when the predictable bouquets arrive, her team members just sigh and congratulate her on having the good sense to marry a woman. Why, they ask plaintively, don't their husbands ever think of such things? The recognition from her coworkers is even more delicious than the flowers.

Another friend reports a well-rehearsed hotel desk routine. In response to the inevitable one-or-two-beds question, she responds, "One," and, without missing a beat, turns to her lover. In her best Bette Davis inflection, she inquires, "Unless, Dahling, there's something you haven't told me." Even potentially hostile outsiders can be disarmed, converted to friendly witnesses when they are invited to share such a charming *entre nous* joke.

Public announcements of special milestones are another means of recruiting witnesses. For one of the threesomes I interviewed, buying a new house was a way of proclaiming their group commitment—if not necessarily their sleeping arrangements—to the world. The sketch on the front of the card tells it all: their closeness and humor and the potential that, at any minute, their family might erupt into a wonderful melee.

Another couple, wanting to put a stop to the buzz of gossip surrounding their relationship, designed a card to

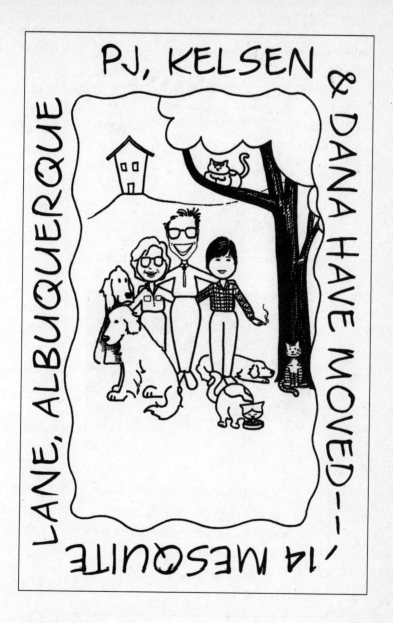

PJ, KELSEN & DANA HAVE MOVED--- '14 MESQUITE LANE, ALBUQUERQUE show friends and family how convivial their twenty-year nonmonogamous arrangement was.

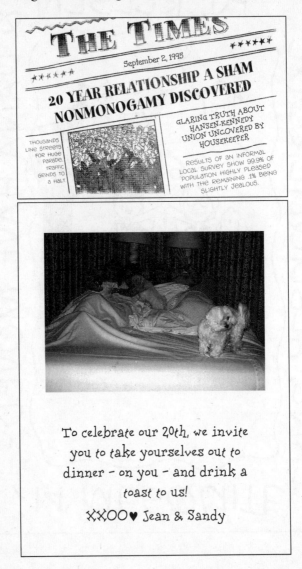

Press releases are another way to recruit relationship witnesses. I was riveted when I came across the following notice in the local gay news:

Martha McPheeters and Marcia Munson have announced their celebration of 21 years of open love, uncommitted sex, firm friendship, and wild adventures. They are organizing an anniversary party on December 10th in Ft. Collins, Colorado. Ironically, Martha and Marcia have never lived together, never dated each other exclusively, nor have they ever been committed to the continuation of their involvement. Theirs could be called an accidental, rather than an intentional, relationship.

With the help of the Ft. Collins telephone directory, I was able to contact Martha and Marcia. They gave me a less abridged version of their curious love story.

Marcia, a wilderness guide, first met her friend and sometimes lover, Martha, when they were both rookie lesbians. For the next two decades, they lived hundreds of miles apart. Whenever they found themselves in the same locale, they would backpack, ski, or bike together. They would also gossip, commiserate about breakups, and sometimes have sex. Chafing at the way their multifaceted relationship seemed less visible to their lesbian friends than more conventional intimacies, they decided to have a noncommitment ceremony to honor their bond. Each was escorted to the celebration by a woman she was currently dating. Marcia started out in a tux, Martha in a satin gown. Halfway through the event they switched out-fits.

An excerpt from their vows reflects the unusual nature of their relationship:

Marcia: Sometimes you have rejected me when I wanted you, you have propositioned me when I was involved elsewhere; and sometimes we have been open to intimacy with each other at the same time. I love you for all those times. In the years I have known you, I have been in three different long-term committed relationships with women I have lived with and loved for years. Today, I know where all three of those women are, and I have warm memories of them, but I'm not as close to any of them, and I don't expect to share real affection with any of them again. With you, Martha, I don't have plans beyond this month—but I expect to share more years of open love, uncommitted sex, firm friendship, and wild adventure. . . .

Martha: Ten years ago, we lived geographically close enough to have one date per week for an entire year. You were a stabilizing influence during this very turbulent period of my life. I discovered you were an excellent confidante. I would and did tell you my hopes and fears, joys and rejections, worries and wonders. Your curious mind, open ears, and warm embraces were instrumental in extricating me from not one but two significant relationships, a job that was destroying me, and a geographic area I found distressingly distasteful. I came to trust you with my emotions, with my mind, and with my body. It was during this period that we defined our love, deciding we could love each other without "falling in love" and that a committed relationship was not for us. We could and would remain uncommitted, sharing love, sex, adventure, and friendship in the moments we found ourselves together.

As a symbol of their liberated yet continuing attachment, Marcia and Martha gave out one hundred gay freedom rings to the assembled guests.

The witnesses for our relationships aren't always drawn from the ranks of the living. Each of the partners in a couple I once worked with in therapy had a close relationship with a gay brother. When the women first met, their brothers were HIV-positive. Over the next five years, each became ill with AIDS and eventually died. The shared experience of caring for their brothers and experiencing each other's grief firsthand deepened the original bond between the two women. On those occasions—holidays and birthdays—when all of them might have gotten together in the past, the partners prepared a special dinner and set the table for four. In two of the places, they placed the boxes that contained their brothers' ashes. They filled their brothers' wine goblets, proposed toasts, and clinked glasses all around. Then they spent the evening reminiscing about all the good times the four of them had had together. They were sure that their brothers, robed in serious angel drag, were smiling on the proceedings from afar.

Breakup Rituals

A year after I attended my first lesbian commitment ceremony, I noticed one of the "brides" browsing nearby in a Berkeley bookstore. She spotted me at the same time, averted her eyes, and left the store quickly. A week later, the news reached me via the grapevine: the newlyweds had decided to dissolve their union. I guessed that the ex-partner who had taken pains to avoid contact with me had been embarrassed that after so much fanfare, things had ended badly for her and her partner.

Our love stories don't always end happily. And if we confine our stories to the happy times, we abdicate the other parts of our lives to embittered ex-lovers or I-told-you-so friends and families or, worse, to the internal witnesses, the voices in our own heads that insist we haven't done it right. No wonder the ex-partner avoided me. She thought that if we talked, I would somehow certify her responsibility for the debacle. She already felt guilty enough.

Shortly after the close encounter with the embarrassed ex I got the following invitation from a different couple:

Ardeth Jenner and Judith Slovak
invite you to witness
their parting at a divorce potluck.
7:00 P.M. Friday, July 7, 1994,
270 West 11th St., New York

LOVERS ARE WONDERFUL BUT EX-LOVERS
ARE FOREVER

After 9 and 1/2 years of partnership we are
formalizing our final transition into friendship with
a gathering of our friends, relations, and neighbors.
Please come help us. We welcome all (civilized)
ideas for ceremony and ritual to mark this passage.

PLEASE NO GIFTS—
not even gifts that could be evenly divided!

Bring: no-fault salad, choosing sides veggie dip,
seven-year-itch watermelon slices, etc.
and don't dress like it's a funeral.

The divorce wasn't exactly a joyful occasion; it was, however, a wonderful alternative to the usual solitary wakes. Instead of shame and invisibility, the exes and their guests swapped stories about rapture and rupture, broken hearts and new awakenings. Late in the evening when I left, I missed the high that I usually feel after a wedding. On the other hand, since I hadn't cried my eyes out, I knew I wouldn't wake up with an emotional hangover.

My first lesbian divorce ceremony also helped me understand a previously inexplicable phenomenon I had witnessed in my own work. Once, after a turbulent session with a dissolving couple, I stuck my head out the window. I was curious to see if they were continuing their donnybrook out on the street. To my amazement, they were strolling away, arms affectionately linked, heads almost touching.

Anyone witnessing such an intimate tête-à-tête would never have believed that ten minutes before, the two lovebirds had been hurling epithets at each other across a chasm of irreconcilable differences.

Acrimonious as such breakup sessions seemed, I realized I was providing separating couples with a face-saving ritual. By agreeing to disagree, and procuring the services of a professional referee, they had demonstrated their honorable intentions toward each other. And Sturm und Drang notwithstanding, they were managing to hammer out the details of the divorce: what to tell respective parents, how to share cat custody, how to divvy up friends and events. Instead of spinning out of control with first one, then the other threatening to jump ship, they were using therapy to leave the relationship with their dignity intact. Their wild whipsawing, in other words, had been stabilized long enough for both to get off the seesaw—albeit their feet barely touched the ground—at the same time. Perhaps most important, the no-fault breakup story they were crafting in the office eliminated the need to blame each other for what had happened. Consequently, they could be amicable outside the office.

Other couples I talked to recruited friends to witness their breakups. Harriet and Cameron, for example, decided to perform their divorce in front of the same group of intimates who had come together for their commitment ceremony. When their friends arrived, the two women explained they wanted to end their relationship formally. Since they were having trouble letting go of each other, they hoped a ritual would help them make the separation they needed to reestablish their independence and ensure that they did not keep slipping back and forth between friend and lover roles.

On the deck where they had uttered their vows a half-dozen years before, they had set out on a table old pieces of pottery, china, flower pots, and other glassware that they said symbolized their "old" relationship. Next to the breakables sat a huge wooden barrel with iron strappings. The assembled guests were instructed to choose any piece of pottery they liked and throw it into the barrel. As it shattered, they were to visualize the severing of the bonds between the dissolving couple. But the guests were also instructed to reflect on their own lives—to imagine that they were breaking ties that held them in relationships or situations from which they wanted to be free.

Hurling crockery with all their might into the barrel, Cameron and Harriet led the way. One by one, the guests joined in. Pow! Crash! Smash! Tinkle. By the time the last piece of crockery was shattered, everyone's face was streaked with sweat and tears. Exorcising the "nice" girls who held on to relationships, things, and feelings proved as cathartic as the two women's original commitment ceremony. Afterward, everyone feasted and then went home exhausted and renewed.

Jane Futcher describes a different sort of dissolution ritual in the anthology *Lesbian Friendships*. When she got together with her first love, Catherine, they had purchased a yellow Honda Civic, which they christened Rubber Ducky. Futcher remembers, "We used to say that Rubber Ducky was our marriage license because the loan—the most money either of us had ever borrowed—was in both our names." Ten years later, Catherine bought out Jane's half of Rubber Ducky. "With that," Jane observes, "our marriage was dissolved."

Karla, another friend, reports that both her major breakup rituals have involved contested property. In the first, she and her partner clustered together all their joint property according to purchase price. Big-ticket items like stereos and couches went in one pile; the toaster, lettuce spinner, lasagna pan (the most hotly contested item) went in another pile, and so forth. After flipping a coin to see who would go first, they took turns going through the piles, selecting the items each preferred. In the second breakup, she went through the same sorting process. Instead of flipping to see who would go first, however, the soon-to-be exes played Chutes and Ladders.

Separation ceremonies are not always amicable or mutual. A lesbian jeweler told me that she was approached by a woman for whom she had originally designed an unusual gold-and-silver commitment ring. The customer asked the jeweler to make a send-up of what such a ring might look like in a semitwisted, half-melted-down state. She hoped when she wore the ring in its new incarnation as a sculpted pendant, it would be noticeable enough to provoke comments. Questions about it would provide the perfect opportunity to describe the origins of the pendant and the betrayal that had ended her partnership.

Rituals for the Uncoupled

Cassandra, an Internet acquaintance, has a beef: because she is uncoupled, no one thinks to give her a few appliances for her kitchen or sheets like couples get during commitment ceremonies. She continues, "I have had to buy everything, while my friends expect me to come up with stuff like that as gifts because they are moving in together. Probably splitting rent and living on a double salary, while I have to manage all the bills on one salary. Why can't we start a nice new tradition of giving these same sort of things for a first apartment?" Before I can respond, she nips my helpful suggestion in the bud.

"Don't tell me to have a housewarming! People bring you really useful stuff like *Jokes for the John* and potted plants."

If coupled dykes are typically invisible, ushered out of existence as soon as their commitment ceremonies are over, imagine the plight of uncoupled lesbians. Without lovers to witness them or partnerships to celebrate, single dykes—their stories untold and unheard—are perpetually on the verge of becoming extinct.

Yet, whether embarking on solo adventures or surrounded by loving friends, the stories of single dykes are also worth telling. Instead of featuring commitments and anniversaries, their tales may showcase accomplishments or special turning points. Everyone would agree that moving to a new apartment or a new country, entering the trying thirties or the sage sixties, finishing a novel or adopting a baby are several events big and brassy enough to earn the spotlight. But noteworthy as they are, such passages are only the barest beginning of opportunities to showcase our lives as uncoupled women. Single lives are rich in change. Transitions happen every month, every week, every moment, if only we care to notice them and give them their due.

For Diana, a determinedly single and celibate friend, every Saturday night marks her hard-won freedom. In the days when she was coupled, she felt most constrained on weekends when she felt obliged to be with her partner. Now she and two other friends (one is even coupled) have agreed to "take back Saturday night." On their "official" group night, they share a meal, review their weeks, gossip, and brainstorm about projects they are working on. It is understood that anyone who dares accept a romantic date on their Saturday night out will be drummed out of the club.

Another friend makes no bones about the fact that her main squeeze is Stonewall, her lab-shepherd mix. Several times a year, she throws a party for Stonewall and his Sunday morning dyke dog-walking group. In true Wegmanesque style, all the four-legged guests are provided their own party hats and favors. Prizes are awarded to the dogs deemed to be most gender dysphoric, most codependent, and most likely to attract a date for its mistress. Games follow the awards ceremony. Besides doggie soccer and Frisbee fetching, there are freestyle events tailored to the rowdier elements in the crowd. Any guests who have not come accompanied by pets are assigned to the cleanup crew.

Jan, another friend, had a hysterectomy five years ago. This year she threw a party to celebrate her cancer-free status. The celebration gave all her friends a chance to fete Jan's continuing presence on planet Earth. Besides collecting all of our verbal tributes, she raised money for her favorite cause. Instead of bringing wine or flowers, everyone was asked to donate money to the local women's cancer resource center. The party netted the organization more than a thousand dollars. Useful as parties are for teasing out those aspects of our lives we consider worth celebrating, such gatherings are not the only way to tell our stories.

One peripatetic friend prefers illustrated newsletters. "Dear friends and family," a recent bulletin begins.

One day while out in the garden, two Wild Canadian Honkers suddenly appeared directly overhead. I had lived in Mendocino eight years and never before seen a wild goose. I took this to be a sign. It was time to head off north. A month later I had my affairs in order, my backpack on my back, Greyhound ticket in hand, and I was headed for Alaska. The wild woman led by the wild goose finally reached the wild land she's been trying to visit for years. I feel like I've come home again.

I lucked out and found a gorgeous house right on the ocean for very little money, which I share with a woman named Laura.

She thinks nothing of camping out in the snow, hiking up the local mountains, ice skating alone at Thimbleberry Lake in the dark with a light on her helmet to show her the way. There are grizzlies here, but Laura never worries about them. Her dog, Goldy, chased a deer through the woods one day, and the deer fell and broke her leg. Laura carried the deer out of the woods alone, realized she couldn't heal her, slaughtered her, and froze the meat for future use, making sure all parts of the deer were used for something. Laura seems to be typical of Alaskans. Am I impressed? You bet.

Perhaps the consummate story of a single lesbian's life transition comes from an almost seventy-year-old friend. Her insouciant take-no-prisoners tale of a well-lived life arrived in the form of a suicide note:

To those I love—

Most of you know that for some time I've been planning to check out—not out of despair of depression—but a desire to end things well.

I've been lucky enough to have had a remarkable life, immeasurably enriched by the love and support of a large (if improbable) group of friends and lovers. I don't want to let it fizzle out in years of debility and dependency. I've gambled enough to know that quitting while you're ahead (or at least even) is wise.

And those of you familiar with my birth date will recognize that the timing of my exit allows me to claim as my epitaph:

TOUJOURS SOIXANTE-NEUF!

Love and good-bye, Sally

The cast of *Rent,* the Tony-winning queer love story currently playing on Broadway, belts out the question again and again: "How do you measure a life? In daylight? In sunsets? In midnights? In cups of coffee? In inches, in miles, in laughter, in strife . . . in truths that she learned or in times that he cried, in bridges he burned, or the way that she died?" At the very same time as our life and death are perfectly mundane events, the lyrics make clear, they are miracles worth celebrating. We are responsible for telling our own stories, singing or dancing them, reciting or drawing them, melting them down or blowing them up, converting them into kisses or collages. We need to perform our stories for one another and anyone else who will listen— and to keep performing them until we stop disappearing from our own lives.

Conclusion: The Way of the Storyteller

"We haven't got any problems."

The buttoned-down butch seconded her girlfriend's opinion with a vigorous nod. "It's true. We're in good shape."

"Really?" I tried not to sound incredulous.

Well, actually, there had been a tiff. Nothing too serious. They just thought it might be good to air their differences in a safe place. "But," the butch added, leaning back and lacing her hands behind her head, "I can't even remember what it was about anymore." She turned to her girlfriend, a carrot-topped elf who was sitting sideways, skinny legs dangling over the arm of the chair. "Can you?"

The elf scratched her head thoughtfully for a moment, then grinned impishly at me. "Nope. I can't remember either."

Still there they were, making themselves at home in my office and waiting expectantly. "Well," I ventured, "as long as you're here, why not just tell me a little about your relationship."

They both beamed. This, I realized, was what they had really come for. They had wanted a witness—someone who would listen to a love story that was indeed extraordinary.

Five years before, the redheaded half of the twosome, Dani, had been diagnosed with melanoma. After conferring with Griff, her partner of seven years, she rejected the recommended regimen of chemotherapy and radiation. Instead, she and Griff turned themselves into an alternative health care research team. They haunted medical libraries and followed up the most improbable leads. Soon Dani was treating herself with everything from shark fin cartilage to visualizations of cancer-gobbling corpuscles muscling their way through her bloodstream.

The cancer hadn't disappeared. But, on the other hand, it hadn't progressed. Dani's doctor was amazed. She had beaten the odds. Dani reached across and squeezed Griff's hand. "I couldn't have done it without her," she said softly. "She's kept me going. I think she's the real cure."

Griff shrugged off the tribute. "I just knew we could do it. Together, we've got this incredible energy."

Faux Ever After: An Ex-Love Story

Often, our relationship stories can make the difference between splitting up and staying together. Perhaps in some cases, they even make the difference between life and death. Considering how vital they are to us, it isn't surprising that we cling to them long after we have declared our partnerships over. Like ghostly presences, these stories often hover on the edge of the cold facts, somewhere beyond the reality of separation.

It's not uncommon for couples who are able to divide beloved pets and favorite CDs nonchalantly to come unglued during negotiations over the photo albums—the illustrated version of their story. Or to remain cucumber cool all through the discussion of giving their landlord notice, only to dissolve into tears at the prospect of announcing their breakup to friends and family. After all, as long as someone believes in it, a love story continues.

When I had first started tracking the Camelot couples, I had been unsure of my role. I vacillated between researcher and advocate, fly on the wall and friend. After they had broken up, however, all ambiguity about my identity ended. I was their chronicler, pure and simple. Perhaps I was the only one who could still detect and relay the faint whisper of their former love stories.

I shuttled back and forth between the exes, listening and, perhaps in some subliminal way, delivering their desperate summonses to each other. When they wept so desolately during our get-togethers, they were communicating indirectly to the absent coauthor of their love story. *Pick up the thread,* they were urging. *Keep it alive.* They scanned my face intently and listened as never before. They were searching for some answer to their plea, some signal that the absent other would indeed start to tell their love story again.

*　　*　　*

At the same time that the partnerships of the Camelot couples were dissolving, my best friend was breaking up with her girlfriend. Whenever I could coax Gail out of the fetal curl on her couch, we would prowl the beaches. And the question, posed over and over, eventually turned into her mantra: Howcouldthishappen? I would try to answer, hazarding a less than flattering appraisal of her ex-lover's character. She would devour every word. And invariably at the end of my effort, there it was again: Howcouldthishappen? It was as though I hadn't spoken at all. I would try again, taking a different tack. This time I might point out her own fatal weakness for femmes who usually dumped her. Again, she listened hungrily.

After the hundredth attempt to explain the inexplicable, I realized it made no difference what I said as long as I answered her. Like a child before bedtime, she was begging: *Tell me a story before the long night begins. You know the sound of her voice and the color of her eyes. Conjure her up for me. Tell me a story. And another. Keep the dark at bay.*

Eventually after hours of combing beaches and histories, we would go our separate ways. She had to endure the long night alone. But the next time we met, it would be there again—the unanswerable question: Howcouldthishappen?

Back and forth. Day after day. Sand and sky. Elaboration and silence. One day during our by now all-too-familiar beach patrols, she chimed in, interrupting me with my own next sentence. And gradually my voice faded to an occasional hmmm, indistinguishable from the surf. When her own voice finally rose above the sound of the waves, I knew she would be okay.

Gradually, Gail came back to life. And, in the process, the forever-after love story that she had clung to for so long finally made way for new tales.

In the beginning, when couples first meet, they tell a story of magical enchantment. After a separation, heartbroken partners begin to retell the tale with a different twist: they had been the victims of sorcery, all right, but the spell they had fallen under had been wicked instead of wonderful. Instead of being rescued from oblivion by that first magic kiss, as they had once believed, they had been snared by it, then by the ten thousand that followed. When the kisses stopped, they were puzzled, then pained, and eventually released. And now they are determined never to be spellbound again.

Perhaps it helps to take long walks by the ocean and have plenty of supportive friends during a breakup. But it is really the story of awakening that cures. Released from the underworld of grief, ex-lovers now portray once-cherished relationships as prisons. And, at long last, they feel free to pursue the dreams they had deferred for years.

Gail began working on a novel that had been lying, untouched, in her desk drawer for years. The day she finished it, she called me up in a state of breathless excitement. She had just met someone new.

Wanted: Wise Women Who've Been There, Done That

I agree to meet Gail and her new love at the annual Butch/Femme Tennis Tournament. As soon as I arrive, Gail rushes up with her new girlfriend in tow—a drop-dead gorgeous six-footer whose caress of a handshake leaves no doubt which side of the net she will play on. Beaming first at her, then at me, Gail declares that her new lover is "wonderful." The furiously blushing girlfriend suddenly feels the need to practice her serve on an empty court. Gail seizes the moment to fill me in.

Lowering her voice to a confidential undertone, Gail whispers, "I'm really in love." She pauses for a few seconds and then adds softly, "It's different this time around. We talk and talk. She's been through a lot, too."

Perhaps I've just witnessed the ultimate storytelling feat: the conversion of breakup pain into new stories—tales that hint at depth and wisdom, while signaling romantic readiness.

Toward the end of her breakup chronicle (the only account of Sapphic sorrows ever penned in iambic pentameter), dyke poet Marilyn Hacker implores her girlfriend not to bury their relationship in a pile of anecdotes. Hacker knows that once she gets filed under "My Last Six Girlfriends: How a Girl Acquires a Past," the affair is over, converted into an ornament. Her ex, decked out in 501s and Forever-After-Foiled-Again stories, will preen before new, admiring eyes and, adorned in the past, will sidle into the future.

Stories and more stories: checkered pasts carefully presented to show potential suitors that we have been done to a fine turn on the rotisserie of life. Winning-the-lottery tales that celebrate the sheer luck of ever finding a soul mate. Breakthrough dramas that sustain us during hard times and cure heartbreak. Our stories are our ceremonies and our witnesses, our marriage licenses and divorce courts, our traditions and our innovations. And most of us perform this magic as effortlessly as we breathe. Yet, what if we trusted our storytelling more? With more skill and confidence, might we be able to turn what is now instinct into an artfully practiced craft?

All Aboard for the Future

At the same tennis tournament, I also ran into Luisa, an ex-client. Luisa, I remembered, had wanted sex; her lover hadn't. As a last resort, they had come to therapy.

Hoping to exorcise the spirits of parents and ex-lovers who seemed to have taken up residence in their bedroom, I had plumbed the histories of each woman in detail. Despite all my probing, nothing shifted. And, to make matters worse, the sensual massage assignments I'd suggested had triggered a whole new round of conflict. Instead of arguing about sex, the two women starting fighting about the exercises. All my efforts fizzled. The partners remained acutely unhappy. Bonded in misery, they were unable to separate and just as unable to stay together. Eventually, they stopped coming to therapy.

When I ran into Luisa at the tournament, I asked what had happened. She told me she and her partner were as unhappy as ever. She was, she murmured, desperate enough to try the remedy that had worked for her Cuban-born parents. She had just made a date to see a *santera*, a fortune-teller.

I remembered how often other clients had come to therapy, admitting a little guiltily that they had seen a psychic or an astrologer. Now a *santera*.

Perhaps because I was off-duty at the tournament, I felt less governed by the rules in effect at the office. Or perhaps I just felt guilty because I had never been able to help Luisa. In any case, I knew that seeing the santera was the right thing to do. For a magical moment, we sat quietly together, not quite sure if we were being bathed by the sun or a ray of hope emanating from somewhere in the future.

The step outside time that Luisa and I shared reminded me of all the other queer time zones hidden by the consensus—a conspiracy really—of clocks. All too well I remembered the insect crawl of pain time, the jerky shuffle of heartbreak recovery, the rewind time of memory, even how during a client's story, time had a way of circling lazily or flashing by so fast it left us both gasping.

The stories of clients and friends existed somewhere outside of clock time. Even my own story had bunched up time like some odd, ungainly carpet that I kept tripping over.

Outside my office, a few weeks before, I had noticed someone strolling toward me. The San Francisco fog, always dense, had been particularly soupy that evening, and it was only after the figure passed under a streetlight that I was able to make her out: stouter, hair more cropped and silvery, but the same dazzling smile. Erin. Ten calendar years. Several lifetimes. A nanosecond. Which was it? How much time had passed since I last had laid eyes on her? I had no idea.

We grabbed a secluded table in a nearby café and began to catch up. She had become a nomad, and I listened, fascinated, as she described her globe-trotting. She listened just as eagerly as I detailed my own emotional voyages. Latte after latte; story after story. Again, I had no idea how much time had gone by. All I knew for sure was that my watch's claim—two hours since we ordered our first round of lattes—was dead wrong.

Story time, unlike clock time, is a zone densely packed with stories: stories stacked up or knotted together in long ropey cords. No matter how contradictory or incongruous, they manage to coexist in this curious zone.

The Way of the Storyteller

Story time is another country: a strange land of many tongues and shifting borders, of peculiar customs and accidental encounters. Perhaps it isn't surprising that such a queer zone would also be the zone of queers.

Coming out happens in story time. The competing stories about who we really are twist time into a pretzel of fast-forward and slow-mo, molasses and zero gravity, past and future. One moment we are egged on at breakneck speed by intimations of heat and mystery, the next slowed to a crawl by the obstacles that go with loving the "wrong" sex.

Coming out may be our first stint in story time, but it's hardly our last. Story time claims us when we fall in love or break up, when we revisit a buried memory or hear some news that shatters life-as-usual. Story time can be thrilling or maddening, wonderful or terrible. And beyond our control.

Most of us feel as though we have no say about the mind-bending adventures that befall us. Shoved or lured by outside forces, we're through the looking glass before we know what happened.

A spin of the cosmic roulette wheel or a high tide of feeling usually lands us in the queer zone. But we *can* follow a less hazardous route into story time. We can storytell our way in.

In order to storytell we have to imagine all the probable and improbable versions of what might happen so vividly that our future visions become a living, breathing part of the present. Storytellers browse regularly among these approximations of reality—tasting, touching, smelling each of them, sensing their texture and heft, trying them on for size, picking favorites, and, when it seems appropriate, convincing others of their merit. Storytellers don't exactly predict what will actually happen, but they do position themselves within range of every imaginable possibility. In short, far from being pawns of fate, storytellers become its midwife.

It would seem that sharing such close quarters with fate might be a risky business. It was reassuring to look up the portentous word in my dictionary. *Fate*, as it turns out, comes from the ever-so-modest root *fari*, which means to be spoken.

To be spoken. No more, no less. Which is exactly what storytellers do. Storytelling is more a matter of chutzpah than clairvoyance—of turning the probable, and even the improbable, into the possible.

Storytelling: Tricks of the Trade

Because peeking into the future has always been mysterious, off-limits to ordinary mortals, we tend to believe that fortune-tellers have some special trick—a particular intuitive talent or, at the very least, some gimmick that enables them to practice their craft. Believing there was indeed a mystery worth unraveling, a group of archaeologists set off a few years ago for Greece. Determined to discover the secret of the famous oracles who plied their trade at Delphi thousands of years ago, the scientists combed archives, hunted for clues at the alleged site of the oracular temple, and talked to the Greek families who could trace their ancestry back for millennia. According to local lore, the priestesses' talents resided in the hallucinogenic properties of a native plant. After ingesting the leaves of the laurel tree, the oracles were reputed to have fallen into a chatty sort of trance.

The archaeologists, being dedicated professionals, immediately set about gathering all the laurel leaves in the vicinity of their digs. They started chewing vigorously. A day passed. Then another. They added fresh leaves to their well-masticated wads of pulp and chewed some more. Despite their zeal, the experiment ended disappointingly. Other than some mild gastrointestinal distress and accompanying burps, there were no other untoward utterances.

Storytelling one's way into story time doesn't require mind-altering substances or special rituals. It simply takes the courage to be inventive, even if it means being contrary. Nothing new for lesbians. Most of us tell multiple and often contradictory stories every day:

- We're queer. We're perfectly normal.
- We live in a straight world. At the same time, we live on another planet.
- Our breakups are the worst thing that ever happened to us. They are the best thing that ever happened to us.

We're already telling stories that fly in the face of logic and common sense. But it's only the beginning. We could tell a lot more.

Stories, Plural

So we're contrarians, against-the-grain mavericks who don't need the trance-inducing drugs and dances, planetary charts, or I-ching coins required by the more conventionally minded soothsayers to leap out of clock time. Nevertheless, we can learn something about the tricks of the trade from experienced fortune-tellers. What is significant about the way the pros practice their craft is not charts or cards, but rather their ability to be alive to multiple stories.

Even though therapists are second-rate sorcerers, they also rely on many stories: fables, called mental disorders, are part and parcel of every therapist's training. No therapist would set up shop without the standard diagnostic manual, a hefty tome that contains descriptions of several hundred personality types. Even the most avid spinner of yarns, working day and night for several lifetimes, couldn't begin to tell all the parables contained in the therapist's bible.

The secret of storytellers of all stripes is simply plenty of stories. And lesbian couples who aspire to storytell their way into story time need to know that forever-after and once-upon-a-time come in all shapes, sizes, and flavors.

At the bus stop. In the sauna. Outside the conference. She is a friend of a friend of a friend. It is a long shot. She is the woman who plowed into the back of our sports car. She is the half-naked juggler at the music festival. She is the woman looking back from the bathroom mirror. She is the new Appaloosa filly. She is on the rebound. She is married. She is a he.

We are repelled. We are impetuous. We are cautious. We are slyly seduced. We are bored. We are the mismatch of the century. We learn a helluva lot.

The combustion is instantaneous. It is a slow burn. Requited, unrequited. Equal, unequal, it lasts a moment, a lifetime; it is a long, smoldering friendship, a fuck-buddy, a soul mate, a secret.

There are plenty of others. Breakups, reunions. She hates the dog. The first grandchild is a pyromaniac. It is an impossible dream, and one day everybody wakes up. It is a group grope. It is a Boston marriage. She died. As far as I'm concerned, she's dead. We are much better friends than lovers. She is family. She is an exquisite memory.

Read these once-upon-a-time and forever-after stories backward and forward, as past and future. Cut them in pieces and give them a good shuffle. Add dozens of others; reshuffle. All these once-upon-a-times and forever-afters coexist, and just like the different cards drawn during a tarot reading, each complicates the story told by the previous card. The stories rub off on one another; they blend, tangle, mutate. To get into story time means having the pluck to tell oneself in. To stay in story time means keeping these stories and many more on the tips of our tongues. Long shots, on the brink of the possible, always on the edge of being told.

A Story About Stories

There is one more story that wise storytellers always tell themselves. It goes something like this: Once upon a time even the most skillful storyteller will come within a hair's breadth of losing her way in story time. Her wits will become so addled that, for a while, she stops being the storyteller and becomes part of the tale.

The tale that proves so hypnotic will go something like this:

> This is noooo story. Hell, no. This is the real thing. Way more powerful than anything you've ever felt or will feel again. Forget everything else. Just relax and let it carry you along.

Or it might go like this:

> No hope left. Utter desolation. May as well be dead.

When the storyteller hears these particular stories, the temptation to abdicate responsibility for telling her own story will be as irresistible as a siren song. But just at the moment she is about to succumb—to lose herself completely—she will remember the hot tip Circe gave Ulysses. And at the very last minute she, too, will remember to lash herself to the mast. She will drift safely past the Sirens back to the sound of her own voice telling her own stories. The end. The beginning.

Marny Hall, Ph.D., is a San Francisco Bay Area psychotherapist with twenty years experience specializing in lesbian relationships. She is the author of *The Lavender Couch: A Consumer's Guide to Psychotherapy for Lesbians and Gay Men,* editor of the anthology *Sexualities,* and contributor to a number of Lesbian anthologies. She lives in Oakland, California with Killer, her philodendron.

Jim Coughenour studied theology at Andover Newton Theological School and the University of Chicago. His cartoons and fiction have appeared in numerous publications and have been featured in several performance pieces. He has also illustrated "Betty & Pansy's Severe Queer Review of San Francisco" and *Crazy Therapies* by Margaret Singer and Janja Lalich (Jossey-Bass). He is the creator of Daimonix Raw Art cards (www.daimonix.com) and a designer with 3 Eye Design+Interactive (www.threeeye.com). At the moment he is at work on the pseudonovel *Doodler,* the café journal of a demented cartoonist.